Digital Health Communications

Technological Prospects and Social Applications Set

coordinated by
Bruno Salgues

Volume 5

Digital Health Communications

Edited by

Benoit Cordelier
Olivier Galibert

iSTE

WILEY

First published 2021 in Great Britain and the United States by ISTE Ltd and John Wiley & Sons, Inc.

ISTE Ltd
27-37 St George's Road
London SW19 4EU
UK

www.iste.co.uk

John Wiley & Sons, Inc.
111 River Street
Hoboken, NJ 07030
USA

www.wiley.com

Library of Congress Control Number: 2021934249

British Library Cataloguing-in-Publication Data
A CIP record for this book is available from the British Library
ISBN 978-1-78630-468-1

MIX
Paper from responsible sources
FSC www.fsc.org FSC® C013604

Contents

Preface

Info-communication Perspectives on Digital Health Communication

As we finalize this collective work, we cannot disregard the health context that is highlighted by the very content of the book. We are confined for public health reasons. Each of us on one side of the Atlantic, like half of the world's population on this day in April 2020, must face the health, social and emotional consequences of the pandemic caused by Covid-19.

We feel the fear of the dangers of disease and the necessary protection of ourselves and our people. We are subjected to a flood of information on the spread of the epidemic in traditional media, as well as on social media, that worries us and sometimes freezes us in fear. We keep in touch with our loved ones via digital tools hardly used by most until now, but which immediately become indispensable to maintain family, friendly and professional links, and at the same time, we are obliged to ensure pedagogical continuity for our students from a distance via digital tools. As actors of these new knowledge mediations, we do so twice over because we must also support our children as they attend their distance courses and evaluations that continue as best as possible during this period.

As you will have understood by reading these lines, the unprecedented health crisis we are experiencing today makes the general issue of the work you are holding in your hands (or reading on a screen) even more topical: how does digital technology contribute to changes in health information and communication? In other words, what are the contemporary challenges of digital communication in health?

The World Health Organization (WHO) defined health in 1946 as "a state of complete physical, mental and social well-being and not merely the absence of disease or infirmity" [OMS 46].

The adjective *health* refers to activities and facilities related to health and hygiene. It takes on a more operational connotation and thus evokes the challenges of public health protection.

In France, a distinction is even made between the social and medico-social sectors – defined by Laws 75-534 for the disabled and 75-535 for social and medico-social institutions, then replaced respectively by Laws 2005-102 and 2002-2 – and the health sector – with Laws 2002-303 on patients' rights and the quality of the health system and 2004-806 for public health policy.

In Quebec, the purpose of Chapter s-2.2 of the Public Health Act is to protect the health of the population and to establish conditions favorable to the maintenance and improvement of the state of health and well-being of the population in general. It is this text that gives the government the authority to declare a state of health emergency, as is the case for the Covid-19 pandemic.

The adjective "*sanitaire*" in French (literally meaning "sanitary" but translated as "health" used adjectivally in English) therefore has a hygienic and operational connotation that may seem more restrictive than the notion of "health". The tensions surrounding this notion are not new: Guillotin and La Rochefoucault-Liancourt were already fighting in 1790 over the absorption of a begging committee by the health committee [EVI 02]. It may be difficult to distinguish between them and we can see that they are part of a continuum between abstraction and concrete practices. For this reason, and without precluding us from continuing our reflections and conceptualization efforts, we use expressions using these words interchangeably here.

Box P.1. *Digital communication in terms of health or digital health communication?*

Covid-19, caused by a coronavirus that has resulted in a global epidemic and an unprecedented wave of hospitalizations for patients with severe acute respiratory syndrome (SARS), is acting as a revealing, even accelerating, force for info-communication issues in the healthcare sector. Plunged into the heart of this health crisis, the world's population is bombarded with journalistic information, as well as strategically targeted communications. In Quebec, during the daily press briefing at 1:00 p.m., François Legault (Premier of Quebec), along with the charismatic Dr. Horacio Arruda (National Director of Public Health) and other members of his cabinet, take stock and give directions for future actions. In France, during the 8 p.m. news, the usual media doctors appear with a myriad of hospital caregivers or epidemiologists who come to testify to the difficulty of coping with the influx of seriously ill patients, the need to remain confined to avoid the spread of an already highly volatile and contagious virus, or the shortage of intensive care beds and protective equipment available to caregivers.

The scientific and institutional expert voice is being solicited as never before, and is relayed or even instrumentalized by political actors in the battle of public opinion being played out in the background. The economic players of the digital society are becoming the universal mediators of a social link that circulates via WhatsApp or TikTok groups. Electronic socialization, which has been completely interwoven into our daily relationships since the massification of global multimedia mobility in the decade 2000–2010, initiated by Steve Jobs and his iPhone in 2008, hegemonically dominates all forms of relationships and information. In this sunny spring, we have resigned ourselves to exchanging and sharing information at a distance, often with humor, about the virus and how to protect ourselves from it: How can we get surgical masks by making them? How can we apply the distancing gestures that protect us from infection? What is the status of tests of promising treatments based on chloroquine or hydroxychloroquine? Are we taking a risk by continuing treatment with cortisone and other anti-inflammatory drugs?

Of course, emotions circulate just as much. Online communities can be formed in a matter of hours, not only within a family or a group of friends, but also within a neighborhood, a street or a building. Just as they serve as a digital foundation or for knowledge sharing between peers, so these communities are inseparable from the gregarious need that drives us: the need to keep in touch with our "local" or "distant" loved ones. Videoconferencing digital platforms are exploding in popularity as we try to maintain our professional activities or reinvent our relationships with family and friends from a distance. Between social, emotional and informational support, digital tools, just like the media of yesteryear, allow us today to create society.

In this spring of 2020, digital communication is everywhere, omnipresent, to the point of obscuring all other channels of mediation. Health issues are central, whether in exchanges on a daily life that reinvented its banality, or on the subject of socio-sanitary issues that were rarely confronted. However, the tensions linked to this massively health-related digital communication have not been swept away – quite the contrary. It would be tempting to give in to a technophilia that was already overwhelming in the past, yet that would be to quickly forget the darker side of the massive use of digital technology.

If we want to return, for example, to the circulation of health information on spaces dedicated to peer-to-peer communication, as all the major generalist social networks are (Twitter, Facebook, Instagram, etc.), the medical profession must face and deny a multitude of fake news stories. Open controversies of a new kind, such as the authorization (by a scientific fringe and a bureaucracy shaken in the temporality of their protocols) of the administration of a treatment not yet approved, are an opportunity for the diffusion in the public space of points of view with no other form of legitimization other than the recognition acquired on the Internet of those who share them.

The broadcasting and digital echo of the debate are part of the new creation of public opinion [CHA 90], which is quick to question any authorized speech. While this phenomenon is not exclusive to the health field, we do see the emergence of lay or amateur expertise [FLI 10]. And what about technological surveillance logics aimed at identifying and preventing, via smartphones, the physical contact of people diagnosed positive for Covid-19 through mobile geolocation applications?

Beyond the "general public" dimension of digital communication in healthcare, medical teams benefit from the creation of true communities of practice [COH 06] that enable them to share crucial knowledge about the disease. However, they are also confronted with the limitations of tools that cannot replace physical interactions, for example, during transmissions between night and day shifts in the hospital environment [GRO 98].

The same is true for local medicine. Although telemedicine allows private practitioners to maintain contact with patients with symptoms of Covid-19, particularly in certain territories already marked by the *medical desert* syndrome, these healthcare professionals nonetheless miss the accuracy of the diagnosis made possible by the traditional face-to-face consultation.

These healthcare professionals are also faced with the rediscovery of a digital divide that was thought to have been reduced by the quality of broadband telecom services, but these services are in fact still unevenly distributed across territories.

As a result, some rural areas, which have not yet been beneficiaries of fiber optic networks, find themselves penalized since videoconferencing services, necessary for remote consultation, require a very high data rate only possible with the installation of fiber.

P.1. The French and Quebec health systems as a heuristic context for analysis

As we will have understood, the spread of Covid-19 and its consequences, medical, economic, social and cultural, constitutes a pivotal moment in contemporary health information and communication issues in a digital context. It brings to the forefront both the consequences of a massive use of digital tools in medical practice and the no less central issues of increasingly digitalized interactions between patients and caregivers, between patients, and between caregivers.

The scope of health communication is therefore very broad. We can try to circumscribe it provisionally in a general definition. From our point of view, health communication encompasses all of the processes involved in creating, disseminating, sharing and evaluating information on health topics that are likely to affect the health of the public, or that are communicated in the organizational context of institutions or professional networks dedicated to health. Digital health communication concerns all health communication phenomena conveyed by sociotechnical information and communication dispositives (SICDs).

It is clear that in 2020, it is deeply illusory to want to dissociate “digital health communication” from a hypothetical “non-digital health communication”. As in all fields of human activity, digital communication is embedded in all forms of interaction and relationships. Nevertheless, it still seems relevant to us to question the specifically digital part of health info-communication issues. Quite simply because we have not yet exhausted our understanding of the consequences of digitization on all of our activities, and particularly in the health sector.

The experience of the Covid-19 health crisis makes this analytical process all the more important since a multitude of supporting discourses are opposed to a no less significant volume of analyses pointing out all the risks inherent in the socio-technical ecosystem. On the one hand, we can identify prescription discourses aimed at the rapid adoption of digital tools facilitating access to information, reducing opportunities for interaction with caregivers or other patients ready to discuss their care pathway, enabling remote medical monitoring or improving the coordination of the action of medical teams [DUP 10, VAL 15]. On the other hand, we can also observe alarmist points of view that indicate the harmful effects of the massive implementation of digital information and communication technologies (DICTs) in terms of the remote monitoring of inhabitants, the development of teleworking that alienates people under the guise of economic optimization, or the future dehumanization of patient care by seeking to digitally compensate for the problem of territorial inequalities in access to care.

The positioning of information and communication sciences in the concert of human and social sciences must allow for relevant, current and heuristic clarifications of approaches to understanding the mechanisms of insertion and, we should also say, of the social insemination of ICT.

Our perspective is anti-deterministic. However, it can well be about the very mechanisms of a deterministic technological thinking at work among critics and promoters of an ever more digital society, increasing or even preserving humanity for some, enslaving it for others. It is at the heart of this tension that the info-communication processes are deployed, between cure and care, which we propose to study in this book. The research carried out for more than 30 years on the specific stakes of the social insertion of DICTs has made it possible to build an active community of researchers who, between the sociology of uses [JAU 11, JOU 00, PER 89], the digital communication of organizations [DUR 09, LEP 02], the new creative and digital industries [BOU 12, MIE 17], the semiotics or semiology of the digital world [BAD 15, BON 13, PIG 09], design [CAR 17b, LEL 02], changes in public debate, the digital mediation of knowledge [JAC 02, MOE 10, PER 12, PER 14] and the challenges of electronic socialization [GAL 05, PRO 00, PRO 06], provide a solid foundation for the identification, analysis and understanding of a digital health society in the making.

The scientific work that gives substance to this approach is located territorially. We question identifiable institutional contexts that, though they are limited to France and Quebec, bring to the forefront issues which, we believe, common to all communities involved in the digitization of health care. However, the health culture is not the same in Canada and France. For example, it is very much marked by the centralizing power of the State in France, and it seems much more imbued with the commitment of healthcare actors in Quebec. The various works presented here will be concerned with showing this context, which seems to us to be rich in similarities, as well as in differences, if only because of their distinct reactions to the logic of the new public management [DEG 14].

Indeed, the idea that corporate management can be applied to all forms of organizations, especially those focused on the common good, such as health organizations, now conditions all activities in the health sector. The logic of efficiency, whose limits are becoming apparent in this period of Covid-19 crisis (e.g. a lack of beds in intensive care units because they are not useful in normal times, a lack of nursing staff because of a decrease in the number of personnel owing to the neoliberal dogma of cost reduction, and a lack of masks, a consequence of the precepts of lean management [BOU 15b], etc.), is predominant in all countries, but with forms of acceptance or resistance that may prove to be different.

It is, of course, the case with regard to the French and Quebec cultural contexts which we focus on here. Similarly, for these two territories, acceptance and resistance to the digitization of care may be similar in many respects, but more specific in others. It seems certain to us, however, that Quebec society and French society can show some form of relevance to reflections on a global health system in crisis; this is a health system in which the care actors, in a form of consensus, question liberal strategic-economic precepts that until now seemed to be the fruit of "vulgar" managerial common sense, despite the exhaustion and repeated alerts of the care workers, particularly in France where half of the emergency services were on strike in September 2019 to demand more resources.

P.2. Information and communication sciences: a theoretical corpus and methodologies for understanding digital communication in healthcare

Without claiming to be exhaustive here, we wish to propose a significant state of the art of digital communication approaches in health led by researchers related or connected to information and communication sciences (ICS).

Numerous works are now available in many HSS disciplines dealing with the analysis of info-communication processes that cross the field of health. In sociology, psycho-sociology, economics and management sciences, researchers are studying the sociotechnical changes that are taking place and that are effective in the mediation between actors and organizations involved in health care. Nevertheless, it seems to us that ICS, because of the elements put forward previously, constitute a very relevant and already rich interdisciplinary base. Indeed, the work presented in this book can draw on a set of empirically proven hypotheses and theories, which are constantly being updated, concerning all the issues of the digital society.

Moreover, the interest in understanding the strategies of actors, which is a key feature of ICS, allows us to take into account macro-social tensions, be they economic or cultural, by linking them, at a meso-level, to individual action logics. In addition, the proximity of ICS research to empirical reality, validated in particular by the numerous partnership research contracts between our laboratories and institutions/organizations in the health sector, testifies to a dynamism in the renewal of problems directly related to the field.

In the same way, the methodological apparatus mobilized can be nourished by various approaches, articulated according to the interdisciplinary affiliations claimed by researchers concerned with not locking their questioning into an overly rigid conceptual straitjacket. As a result, cross methodologies, mainly articulating qualitative approaches in a comprehensive perspective, are deployed. This will be a question of finely perceiving the logics of actions via semi-directed interviews, as well as of strongly mobilizing ethnographic approaches of the Internet [JOU 13]; the semio-pragmatic analysis of site design can also be used [ODI 11], as can the analysis of online discourse [MAR 16].

P.3. For a critical approach to digital health communication

While we do not wish to further evoke here the multiplicity of empirical approaches practiced in digital communication, it seems to us necessary to mention the main currents of communicational thinking in health. We believe that all of them are defined by a critical distance towards supporting discourses or organizational projects that aim to make ICTs the all-encompassing solutions to most, if not all, of the health sector problems. This critical distance, the result of observations made as closely as possible to the uses and info-communication practices of patients and caregivers, never precludes an increase in generality involving a systemic questioning of the dominant neoliberal perspectives.

It is in this perspective that Dominique Carré and Jean-Guy Lacroix, in a Franco-Quebec approach that is very similar to ours today, aimed to understand in a general and global way the societal stakes of the computerization of care. Not exclusively focused on organizational issues, their approaches jointly see the beginnings of a mutation of expertise and a technician ideology promoting the empowerment of a patient who is supposed to become an actor of his or her care… online. It is then a question of evaluating the effects of the "computer transplant" [CAR 01b] in a constantly changing health sector, between renewed regulations, major industrial and economic stakes and the imposition of new rationalizing managerial standards. The objective of the two authors is clear: to show the role of communicating information technology in the dual process of merchandizing and managerialization underlying the "outpatient shift"; the latter aiming to reduce the overall costs of hospital care considered too expensive.

The research conducted or highlighted by Carré and Lacroix questions the promotion of sociotechnical empowerment aimed at encouraging patients to co-produce the care they receive by automating part of the medical follow-up [CAR 01a]. They prefigure all or part of the work that we now refer to as "digital communication in health". Since then, these perspectives have not only been largely updated, but also constitute a particularly lively research subject within the ICS. As a result of the pioneering approach of these two authors, health studies will attract the interest of a growing number of ICS researchers, providing empirical support for the major theoretical currents in our discipline. This work repeatedly questions the issues of the digitalization of today; the field of healthcare is a central terrain for exploring the developments of the digital society. We propose a synthetic panorama of this field in the following sections.

P.4. Digital health communication in the workplace

As an extension of the issues defined by Carré and Lacroix, work on digital communication for health organizations is very much alive in the French-speaking ICS community. It highlights the limits of information technology in health care, obviously at the level of institutions, as well as at the level of so-called "urban" professional practices. In particular, following the initial work claiming a crossover between health and organizational communication [GRO 99], and short of the work aiming to cover the entire problematic field, where computerization is supported by an increasingly commercial logic, as well as an industrial one [SAL 16], the work carried out in digital communication of organizations is focused on more limited areas.

From a critical perspective, they highlight the rationalization processes brought about by the application of neo-management in healthcare institutions [BAZ 08, BON 05] and the increasing computerization of patient care processes by healthcare professionals. In a neoliberal context marked by the disengagement of the State and the need to reduce costs, the implementation of the personalized medical record is an emblematic example [MAY 12]. Rationalization processes, aimed at making healthcare ever more efficient, are then nourished by the monitoring and control possibilities offered by digital technologies. The same applies to services based on quantified self or digital self-measurement, which are becoming widespread via smartphone applications. These applications encourage Internet or mobile users to share their personal health data (e.g. the number of calories they spend on their morning jog) with their online community. The aim is to evaluate a positive or even negative physiological progression or evolution, such as weight gain. This measurement of physiological performance, calibrated to that of other members of the community [ARR 13], reflects a form of cybernetic self-optimization, which is certainly fun, but which reminds us of the automation logic already identified by Dominique Carré in 2001. Moreover, these practices, conveyed by industrial players in the collaborative web economy [BOU 10], reinforce the need to establish and respect a "data ethic". Indeed, what about the marketing exploitation of individual information concerning intimacy? What can be said about the possible risks of using these data [BER 14], for example, by banking institutions looking for reliable information to establish the insurance rate of a mortgage loan?

On another level, following in particular the above-mentioned work of Anne Mayère, recent research points to tinkering and other misuse of the system by healthcare personnel who refuse to accept the increased bureaucracy induced by the traceability of acts and procedures; traceability that is essentially digital ("paperless" logic) and strongly linked to the implementation of the famous electronic personal medical record [COR 13, GRA 17]. From the same perspective, Luc Bonneville and Sylvie Grosjean attempt to explore digital communication in health as the product of a paradoxical opposition between two social logics: the emancipatory logic of promoting a professional practice free of low added value tasks, in favor of time spent with the patient and/or improving care ("clinical reason"), and the reifying logic of a computerization ratio that standardizes professional practices with a permanent concern for efficiency ("economic reason"), leaving caregivers with no other choice than to bypass them with "tinkered" substitution devices [BON 07].

In the wake of questions concerning the meso info-communication approach of health organizations, work is focusing more specifically on groups or categories of healthcare professionals affected by digital technology, or even emerging through digital mediations. How does digital communication accompany the profound changes in the organization of care in healthcare institutions, outside of hospitals and other clinics, or in networks trying to optimize interprofessional coordination in territories with unequal health resources [BOU 03]? The aim here is to show the emergence of new forms of professionalism based on the "scientific" and "operational" mediation of medical knowledge. As a result, new digital healthcare professions are emerging, using the Internet to create communities of patients led either by healthcare professionals switching to community management or by community managers trained in the specificities, particularly ethical, of digital communication in health [GAL 14].

P.5. Digital communication in health: between strategic communication, public space and empowerment

As a result, between understanding the uses, non-uses and misuses of ICT in the workplace, support for the managerial rationalization of healthcare teams and new professionalization, research into digital communications in healthcare organizations provides an original insight into the challenges of the sector. However, thinking about persuasive digital communication produced by healthcare organizations and professionals cannot be limited to communication at work.

Emerging approaches are also questioning the communication strategies implemented by institutions, independently of the communication of prevention authorities. In an info-communication environment marked by a form of mistrust, or even distrust, of the institutional discourse [PAR 15], this is a question of providing the clearest possible information to make the patient a (convinced) stakeholder in the quality of care. Although this information is massively transmitted via the Internet, public hospitals, particularly in France, are constrained by data security standards not to develop the "communication" function in organizational charts. This results in the dissemination of very practical, not to say administrative, top-down information, which cannot compete with participative and collaborative general public health information systems, such as Doctissimo. This strategic approach to communication in public health establishments [AMB 18] highlights the role of the Internet in the construction of true "hospital brands" [MED 11]. At the edge of the digital communication of organizations, this is indeed a more rooted form of digital public health communication.

An important part of the digital health communication work carried out in ICS is questioning online public communication. In a dominant paradigm of promoting *health democracy* and the empowerment of a patient who must become an actor in his or her care, the research conducted here attempts to analyze the different communication strategies orchestrated by public authorities towards the general public. The Internet then feeds the imagination of a recomposed public space in which the patient and his or her caregivers ideally participate in the public health debate and dedicated political decisions. Paradoxically enough, this research shows that the logic of a persuasive public advertising communication, in which the patient is a target to be convinced, is resistant to disappear in favor of a more "collaborative" approach, which is nevertheless desired. In a perspective marked by health promotion, despite the objective of going beyond "traditional" communication strategies, public authorities often consider that

> "the other" is not an enigma to be deciphered or discovered, but a stranger who must be convinced so that he will modify or change his attitude. [REN 07]

The same applies to the work of the ComSanté team, which is continuing and diversifying this approach [KIV 09]. This research resonates with other works that highlight attempts at the dialogical adaptation of health institutions, particularly in the face of health crises. In the context of the massification of SICDs specific to the collaborative Web, the controversies arising from these crises are deployed in digital public debate arenas in which the biomedical voice is challenged [OLL 15], or at least discussed, either by Internet users with no particular knowledge of the disease other than experiential knowledge, or by citizens who want to make their voices heard, often critical and discordant, on crisis management.

Digital public health communication continues to be in tension between the strategies of institutional, political and industrial actors and the more informative and community-based logics aimed at emancipating all citizens through knowledge and reasoned and reasonable discussion. Public authorities are forced to completely review their communication policies, giving priority to participatory mechanisms in order to play an active role in a health public space [PAI 07], which must nevertheless be controlled. It is therefore a question for ICS researchers to understand the new modalities of a strategic communication called 2.0 which, under the guise of a health democracy aiming at the participation of all in the improvement of health care, would seek to better orient exchanges in a logic oscillating between political communication and therapeutic education [ROM 10].

The patient-actor becomes the pivot of this new info-communicational strategy. No longer just a passive receiver of public health info-communication campaigns, the patient uses SICDs to participate in the improvement of care, or even to co-create therapeutic innovation. This is how very recent research is studying how the patient is projected at the heart of the creation of e-health solutions [BON 19]. The perspective is perfectly summarized by Marc Lemire. For the Canadian researcher, the use of the Internet immediately implies a proactive approach on the part of the patient. For Lemire,

> this attitude differs from passive obedience, an attitude usually attributed to the patient and generally expected in "classic" models of healthcare management. This is the case with the professional model of compliance, which remains widespread in modern healthcare systems. [LEM 09]

However, not all citizens, potential users of health care, are equally equipped to deal with a digital divide that may, in the long term, create real health information disparities. Indeed, as Joëlle Kivits and Sophie Gendarme point out, access to health information no longer seems to be an economic or technological issue, but a question of health literacy, that is, the ability to

> understand media content (Rootman, Gordon-El-Bihbety, 2008), an ability that is more important for people with higher levels of education. In this sense, it is a marker of inequality in terms of Internet use, and more generally in terms of health. [KIV 15]

P.6. Digital health communication: the promise of cognitive, social and emotional support

The massification of digital tools is therefore profoundly modifying the informational and communicational practices of patients and their caregivers. These practices seem to be deeply emotional, on the one hand, because of the need to be informed about our pathology or that of a loved one, to better understand the treatment and its side effects, and to grasp the issues at stake in terms of duration or hospital/outpatient care and, on the other hand, because of the need to share our experience and benefit from that of others in the face of a disease.

Work on online patient information modalities is still relevant, systematically reactivating the analysis of tensions and struggles for recognition between knowledge from the experience of care and knowledge from scientific and academic institutions. This is how Viviane Clavier highlights a form of unpreparedness on the part of healthcare professionals in the face of general questions related to current events asked by patients, which lead the specialist into non-specific answers for which she or he will have a form of natural distrust [CLA 19]. This is why health information is consulted, discussed, shared and produced by patients who are concerned about better understanding of the disease, its treatment and, above all, how daily life will be organized around it in the future. Marc Lemire encourages the academic community to consider with great interest this "heterodox knowledge" that resonates or competes with "biomedical knowledge" [LEM 09]. So-called lay knowledge, although it can compete with institutionalized biomedical hegemony in the context of a rebalanced patient–professional care relationship [ACK 10], nonetheless remains a fully-fledged informational and emotional resource for patients. As noted by Pierre Mignot and Dorsaf Omrane in their study of a digital breast cancer prevention dispositive, it is necessary to underline "the persuasive power of 'knowledge from experience' in the spaces of online exchanges between the people concerned" [MIG 18].

This new form of experiential expertise [PAG 14] constitutes, at a time when the expert patient is becoming a professional, a central subject of study that we will find in Chapters 7 and 8 of this book. This new cognitive and informational situation is also coupled with a significant social and emotional contribution. If the patient's presence online is motivated by the need to be informed, it is also an opportunity to forge links with other patients who share a similar reality. This is how online social and emotional support [CHE 19] constitutes the other side of a digital community link whose social logic has yet to be widely explored in the health sector.

P.7. And finally, how can we take care of digital workers?

To conclude this overview of digital communication in health from the point of view of ICS, we would like to reiterate that the digital is itself considered a major health issue, especially at work [BOU 15a]. The idea here could be similar to the perspectives opened up by Bernard Stiegler in his pharmacology of the digital world [STI 06], where online practices are both a remedy for many informational and relational deficiencies, as well as a social poison. The aim here is to understand the psycho-sociological risks linked in particular to what we could define as "connective burn-out". Some researchers in the field therefore favor the term techno-sociological risks (TSR) such as

> all the physical and psychological disorders incurred by an employee, as soon as he or she becomes part of a work situation where information and communication technologies (ICT) play a central role in the accomplishment of his or her missions. [OLI 19]

In the case of a strong dematerialization of the activity in what is commonly today called digital labor [CAR 15], workers, whether they are members of the "pronetariat" according to the terminology of the futurologist Joël de Rosnay [DER 06] or representatives of a hyper-connected management [CAR 17a, CAR 19], suffer from the impossibility of extracting themselves from the platformized digital pressure (e.g. in the case of self-employed workers who have been uberized and enslaved by the uninterrupted process of online orders) or managerial (e.g. the obligation for a community manager to remain on the lookout for posts that negatively affect the image of his or her employer on social networks) [HAS 19].

P.8. Diagnosis and treatment

Digital technology continues to transform our society. It is even helped by a completely organic virus. An unlikely alliance, but how terribly effective. We now leave you with this book and these explorations to continue thinking about the changes that are taking place.

Olivier: "We'll talk again to write the introduction, but now I have to leave you. I have a call about one of my students' thesis."

Benoit: "Excellent. That gives me a few moments to prepare for my videoconference consultation with my proctologist. See you tomorrow!"

Olivier GALIBERT
University Burgundy Franche-Comté
Benoit CORDELIER
University of Quebec in Montreal (UQAM)

Dijon/Montreal, March 2021

P.9. References

[AMB 18] AMBROSINI C.-F., La communication hospitalière publique à l'ère digitale, Information and Communication Sciences Thesis, Université de Nice Sophia Antipolis, Nice, 2018.

[ARR 13] ARRUABARRENA B., QUETTIER P., "Des rituels de l'automesure numérique à la fabrique autopoïétique de soi", *Les Cahiers du numérique*, vol. 9, no. 3, pp. 41–62, 2013.

[BAD 15] BADULESCU C., "La communication numérique en terrain sensible", *Questions de communication*, no. 28, pp. 81–100, 2015.

[BAZ 08] BAZET I., JOLIVET A., MAYERE A., "Pour une approche communicationnelle du travail d'organisation : changement organisationnel et gestion des événements indésirables", *Communication & Organisation*, no. 33, pp. 30–39, 2008.

[BER 14] BÉRANGER J., BOUADI R., "Approche éthico-juridique de l'usage des données médicales à caractère personnel", *Les Cahiers du numérique*, vol. 10, no. 2, pp. 93–123, 2014.

[BON 05] BONNET J., "Interprofessionnalité et complexité : une tentative de compréhension et d'articulation des cultures et des pratiques professionnelles liées à la santé", in AUBERT M. (ed.), *Interprofessionnalité en gérontologie*, Érès, Toulouse, 2005.

[BON 13] BONACCORSI J., "Chapitre 6 – Approches sémiologiques du web", in BARATS C. (ed.), *Manuel d'analyse du web en Sciences Humaines et Sociales*, Armand Colin, Paris, 2013.

[BOU 03] BOURRET C., "La santé en réseaux", *Études*, vol. 399, no. 9, pp. 175–189, 2003.

[BOU 10] BOUQUILLION P., MATTHEWS J.-T., *Le web collaboratif mutations des industries de la culture et de la communication*, Presses universitaires de Grenoble, Grenoble, 2010.

[BOU 12] BOUQUILLION P., *Creative economy, creative industries : des notions à traduire*, Presses universitaires de Vincennes, Saint-Denis, 2012.

[BOU 15a] BOUDOKHANE-LIMA F., FELIO C., "Les usages professionnels des TIC : des régulations à construire", *Communication & Organisation*, vol. 48, no. 2, pp. 139–150, 2015.

[BOU 15b] BOUVILLE G., TREMPE C., "La mise en place du lean management. Un bouleversement de l'univers hospitalier ?", in FERMON B. (ed.), *Performance et innovation dans les établissements de santé*, Dunod, Paris, 2015.

[CAR 01a] CARRÉ D., "À la frontière du marchand et du non marchand. Place des téléservices dans la réorganisation du secteur de la santé", *Études de communication*, vol. 23, no. 1, p. 3, 2001.

[CAR 01b] CARRÉ D., LACROIX J.G., *La santé et les autoroutes de l'information. La greffe informatique*, L'Harmattan, Paris, 2001.

[CAR 15] CARDON D., CASILLI A., *Qu'est-ce que le digital labor ?* INA, Bry-sur Marne, 2015.

[CAR 17a] CARAYOL V., *La laisse électronique : les cadres débordés par les TIC*, MSHA, Pessac, 2017.

[CAR 17b] CARDOSO S., BOURDAA M., "Design et transmedia : projet, expérience usager, worldbuilding au cœur des disciplines SHS", *Revue française des sciences de l'information et de la communication*, no. 10 [Accessed 23 April 2020], 2017.

[CAR 19] CARAYOL V., LABORDE A., "Les organisations malades du numérique", *Communication & Organisation*, vol. 56, no. 2, pp. 11–17, 2019.

[CHA 90] CHAMPAGNE P., *Faire l'opinion le nouveau jeu politique*, Éditions de Minuit, Paris, 1990.

[CHE 19] CHERBA M., THOËR C., TURBIDE O. *et al.*, "Le soutien social en ligne comme mode d'intervention psychosociale : revue de littérature, pistes de recherche et recommandations pour les intervenants", *Santé Publique*, vol. 31, no. 1, pp. 83–92, 2019.

[CLA 19] CLAVIER V., "La place de l'information dans les pratiques professionnelles des diététiciennes : au croisement des missions d'éducation, de prévention et de soin", *I2D – Information, données & documents*, pp. 114–133, 2019.

[COH 06] COHENDET P., CREPLET F., DUPOUËT O., *La gestion des connaissances firmes et communautés de savoir*, Économica, Paris, 2006.

[COR 13] CORDELIER B., "Mise en invisibilité des individus et reconnaissance des activités", *Communication et organisation*, no. 44, pp. 29–40, 2013.

[DEG 14] DE GAULEJAC V., *La société malade de la gestion idéologie gestionnaire, pouvoir managérial et harcèlement social*, Le Seuil, Paris, 2014.

[DER 06] DE ROSNAY J., *La révolte du pronétariat*, Fayard, Paris, 2006.

[DUR 09] DURAMPART M., "Les TIC dans les organisations : des partenaires difficiles à contrôler", *Hermès, La Revue*, vol. 54, no. 2, pp. 221–227, 2009.

[EVI 02] EVIN C., *Les droits des usagers du système de santé*, Berger-Levrault, Paris, 2002.

[FLI 10] FLICHY P., *Le sacre de l'amateur sociologie des passions ordinaires à l'ère numérique*, Le Seuil, Paris, 2010.

[GAL 13] GALIBERT O., "L'injonction participative au débat environnemental en ligne : imaginaires d'Internet, démocratie environnementale et communication engageante", *Les enjeux de l'information et de la communication*, vol. 14, no. 1, pp. 35–49, 2013.

[GAL 14] GALIBERT O., "Approche communicationnelle et organisationnelle des enjeux du Community Management", *Communication & Organisation*, no. 46, pp. 265–278, 2014.

[GRO 98] GROSJEAN M., LACOSTE M., "L'oral et l'écrit dans les communications de travail, ou les illusions du 'tout écrit'", *Sociologie du travail*, no. 4, 1998.

[GRO 99] GROSJEAN M., LACOSTE M., *Communication et intelligence collective*, PUF, Paris, 1999.

[GRO 07] GROSJEAN S., BONNEVILLE L., "Logiques d'implantation des TIC dans le secteur de la santé", *Revue française de gestion*, vol. 172, no. 3, pp. 145–157, 2007.

[GRO 19] GROSJEAN S., BONNEVILLE L., REDPATH C., "Le patient comme acteur du design en e-santé : design participatif d'une application mobile pour patients cardiaques", *Sciences du design*, vol. 9, no. 1, pp. 65–83, 2019.

[HAS 19] HASSANI N., "Hyperconnexion des Community Managers : injonction ou propension ?", *Communication & Organisation*, vol. 56, no. 2, pp. 93–107, 2019.

[JAC 02] JACQUINOT-DELAUNAY G., "Au-delà du modèle canonique de la relation maître-élève : les TIC ou comment faire circuler les signes de la présence", in GUIR R. (ed.), *Pratiquer les TICE, former les enseignants et les formateurs à de nouveaux usages*, De Boeck, Brussels, 2002.

[JAU 11] JAUREGUIBERRY F., PROULX S., *Usages et enjeux des technologies de communication*, Érès, Toulouse, 2011.

[JOU 00] JOUËT J., "Retour critique sur la sociologie des usages", *Réseaux*, vol. 100, no. 2, pp. 487–521, 2000.

[JOU 13] JOUËT J., LE CAROFF C., "Chapitre 7 – L'observation ethnographique en ligne", in BARATS C. (ed.), *Manuel d'analyse du web en Sciences Humaines et Sociales*, Armand Colin, Paris, 2013.

[KIV 09] KIVITS J., LAVIELLE C., THOËR C., "Internet et santé publique : comprendre les pratiques, partager les expériences, discuter les enjeux", *Santé Publique*, vol. 21, pp. 5–12, 2009.

[KIV 15] KIVITS J., GENDARME S., "8 – Les institutions publiques, Internet et la santé : de l'offre publique aux usages privés", in MEIDANI A. (ed.), *La santé : du public à l'intime*, Presses de l'EHESP, Rennes, 2015.

[LAF 07] LAFON B., PAILLIART I., "Malades et maladies dans l'espace public", *Questions de communication*, no. 11, pp. 7–15, 2007.

[LEM 09] LEMIRE M., "Internet et responsabilisation : perspective de l'usager au quotidien", *Santé Publique*, vol. 21, pp. 13–25, 2009.

[LEP 02] LEPINE V., "Une entreprise sidérurgique aux prises avec le groupware : apports d'une étude empirique", *Les enjeux de l'information et de la communication*, no. 1, pp. 65–74, 2002.

[LEP 13] LEPINE V., PARENT B., "De la visibilité à l'individuation des cadres hospitaliers : l'obstacle de la dyschronie", *Communication & Organisation*, vol. 44, no. 2, pp. 41–52, 2013.

[MAR 16] MARCOCCIA M., *Analyser la communication numérique écrite*, Armand Colin, Paris, 2016.

[MAY 12] MAYERE A., BAZET I., ROUX A., "'Zéro papier' et 'pense-bêtes' à l'aune de l'informatisation du dossier de soins", *Revue d'anthropologie des connaissances*, vol. 6, no. 1, pp. 115–139, 2012.

[MEA 10] MEADEL C., AKRICH M., "Internet, tiers nébuleux de la relation patient-médecin", *Les Tribunes de la santé*, vol. 29, no. 4, pp. 41–48, 2010.

[MED 11] MEDINA AGUERREBERE P., "La diffusion online de la marque hospitalière : le cas des hôpitaux français", *Quaderni*, no. 74, pp. 97–104, 2011.

[MIE 17] MIEGE B., *Les industries culturelles et créatives face à l'ordre de l'information et de la communication*, Presses universitaires de Grenoble, Grenoble, 2017.

[MOE 10] MOEGLIN P., *Les industries éducatives*, PUF, Paris, 2010.

[ODI 11] ODIN R., *Les espaces de communication. Introduction à la sémio-pragmatique*, Presses universitaires de Grenoble, Grenoble, 2011.

[OLI 19] OLIVERI N., PELISSIER N., "Repenser les dispositifs numériques des organisations au prisme des risques technosociaux (rts), identification, évaluation, prévention", *Les Cahiers du numérique*, vol. 15, no. 4, pp. 87–111, 2019.

[OLL 15] OLLIVIER-YANIV C., "La communication publique sanitaire à l'épreuve des controverses", *Hermès, La Revue*, vol. 73, no. 3, pp. 69–80, 2015.

[OUM 18] OUMRANE D., MIGNOT M., "Préventions des cancers du sein : ce que la controverse fait à l'action publique", *Les enjeux de l'information et de la communication*, vol. 19, no. 3, pp. 41–55, 2018.

[PAG 14] PAGANELLI C., CLAVIER V., "S'informer via des médias sociaux de santé", *Le temps des médias*, no. 23, winter, 2014.

[PAR 16] PARRINI-ALEMANNO S., "Chapitre 12 – Recomposition organisationnelle à l'aune de la confiance généralisée : l'exemple des Institutions de soins en France", in DELAYE R. (ed.), *La confiance : relations, organisations, capital humain*, EMS Éditions, Caen, 2016.

[PER 89] PERRIAULT J., *La logique de l'usage essai sur les machines à communiquer*, Flammarion, Paris, 1989.

[PER 12] PERAYA D., MARQUET P., HÜLSMAN T. *et al.*, "Médiation, médiations…", *Distances et médiations des savoirs*, no. 1 [Accessed 22 January 2014], 2012.

[PIG 09] PIGNIER N., "Sémiotique du webdesign : quand la pratique appelle une sémiotique ouverte", *Communication & Langages*, vol. 159, no. 1, pp. 91–110, 2009.

[PRO 00] PROULX S., LATZKO-TOTH G., "La virtualité comme catégorie pour penser le social : l'usage de la notion de communauté virtuelle", *Sociologie et sociétés*, vol. XXXII, no. 2, pp. 99–122, 2000.

[PRO 06] PROULX S., *Communautés virtuelles penser et agir en réseau*, Les Presses de l'université Laval, Quebec, 2006.

[REN 07] RENAUD L., RICO DE SOTELO C., "Communication et santé : des paradigmes concurrents", *Santé Publique*, vol. 19, pp. 31–38, 2007.

[ROM 10] ROMEYER H., *La santé dans l'espace public*, Presses de l'EHESP, Rennes, 2010.

[SAL 16] SALGUES B., *Health Industrialization*, ISTE Press Ltd, London and Elsevier Ltd, Oxford, 2016.

[STI 07] STIEGLER B., "Questions de pharmacologie générale. Il n'y a pas de simple pharmakon", *Psychotropes*, vol. 13, no. 3, pp. 27–54, 2007.

[VAL 15] VALLANCIEN G., *La médecine sans médecin. Le numérique au service du malade*, Gallimard, Paris, 2015.

Acknowledgments

We would like to warmly thank Bruno Salgues, in charge of the "Technological Prospects and Social Applications" Set at ISTE Group, for his advice, his proofreading and his patience in the writing and editing process.

This book is the culmination of years of efforts and collaborations, exchanges, study days at UQAM and the University Burgundy Franche-Comté, and symposiums within the ACFAS (*Association francophone pour le savoir*) and ICA (International Communication Association) congresses. We would like to thank the researchers with whom we exchanged views on these occasions. In particular, we would like to thank Sylvie Parinni Alemanno of the DICEN-IDF laboratory (CNAM) and Christine Thoër, former director of ComSanté, as well as their teams, for their valuable logistical and financial contributions to the organization of the "Organization, Digital Health" study days in 2017.

The entire project would also not have been possible without the unwavering support of the French, Canadian and Quebec funding agencies that support our research teams. For CIMEOS (EA 4177) and the LIPSTIC laboratory of excellence: the *Agence nationale de la recherche* (Labex LipSTIC, ANR-11-LABX-0021), the Burgundy-Franche-Comté Region and the European Regional Development Fund. For the ComSanté research center: the Social Sciences and Humanities Research Council (SSHRC), the *Fonds de recherche du Québec – Société et culture* (FRQSC), the *Conseil de la recherche et de la création* (COREC, UQAM).

Acknowledgments written by Benoit CORDELIER and Olivier GALIBERT.

Author Biographies

Pénélope Codello

Pénélope Codello, PhD, is a professor at HEC Montréal. Her research and teaching focus on soft skills and personal development; her work also focuses on education sciences and managerial perspectives. Codello is interested in the analysis of social cohesion in leadership development and is also a Gestalt coach. Finally, she also exercises major responsibilities in the educational and administrative management of her school.

Benoit Cordelier

Benoit Cordelier is a professor in the department of Social and Public Communication at Université du Québec à Montréal (UQAM), where he is a researcher at the *Centre de recherche sur la communication et la santé* (ComSanté) and at the Chair of Public Relations and Marketing Communication. Cordelier is also editor of *Communiquer*, a social and public communications journal. His research focuses on change and organizational processes, as well as the communicational aspects of culture in online consumer communities.

Damien De Meyere

Damien De Meyere is a linguist, computer scientist and PhD student at the *Institut langage et communication* of the Université catholique de Louvain (Belgium). De Meyere specializes in the development of natural language processing software which enables textual productions from socio-digital platforms to be analyzed. His research focuses on the use of information extraction techniques in order to establish a typology of lay expertise within health forums such as Doctissimo.

Stéphane Djahanchahi

Stéphane Djahanchahi is a PhD student at the Université de Bourgogne Franche-Comté under the supervision of Olivier Galibert and Benoit Cordelier. His research focuses on the Health Knowledge Innovation research axis (*Santé savoirs innovation*, 2SI) of the CIMEOS laboratory and Labex LipSTIC. His thesis focuses on the organization and instrumentalization of online communities, the theme being therapeutic cannabis. Djahanchahi's research themes are the construction of expertise within online communities and methods of legitimizing knowledge used by some of their members.

Olivier Galibert

Olivier Galibert is an Information and Communication Sciences professor at the Université de Bourgogne Franche-Comté. Director of the CIMEOS laboratory, his research questions the forms of community socialization at work on the Internet and as well as Intranets. Today, his investigations are centered on community management issues in communities of patients, caregivers and health professionals.

Géraldine Goulinet Fité

Géraldine Goulinet Fité is a doctor in Information and Communication Sciences at the Université Bordeaux Montaigne. Associated with the MICA laboratory (*Médiation information communication art*), she participates in work on vulnerability within the axis of organization communication and society. Goulinet Fité's research focuses on the contribution of digital uses in health, regarding the ethical and practical exercise of home care in the context of aging and chronic disease.

Anne Mayère

Anne Mayère is a professor at the Université Paul Sabatier Toulouse 3, and a researcher at the CERTOP laboratory, UMR CNRS, jointly responsible for the Santal axis. Her research, with a basis in the communication of organizations, focuses on the rationalization of information production and communication activities, such as that employed in different organizations, and in particular in health organizations.

Mayère's current research programs relate to developments in e-health and Big Data in health.

Pierre Mignot

Pierre Mignot is a lecturer in Information and Communication Sciences at the *Laboratoire d'études et de recherches appliquées en sciences sociales* (LERASS) of Université de Toulouse 3 – Paul Sabatier. His research focuses on representations in the context of health and prevention. Mignot completes analyses of discourses and content from social media including Facebook and Twitter, but more particularly on the practices of health practitioners and the population concerned with cancer prevention and screening.

Laurent Morillon

Laurent Morillon is a professor at the Université des Antilles, pôle Martinique, where he is a researcher at LC2S (UMR 8053). Joint head of the Org&Co study and research group of the SFSIC[1], his research focuses on the epistemological practices and models of actors in an organizational context, notably researchers in organizational communication and communicators.

David Morquin

David Morquin is a doctor and specialist in internal medicine and infections at the Centre hospitalier universitaire de Montpellier, where he manages the delegation for the use of digital technology, which he created. In 2019, he defended his PhD in management sciences (information systems) on the use of electronic health records in public hospitals. Morquin's current research themes are digital transformation among professional workers, the impacts of computerization on medical reasoning and clinical practices.

Ewan Oiry

Ewan Oiry is a professor of human resources management at the École des sciences de gestion – Université du Québec à Montréal (ESG-UQAM). His current research themes include skills management, HRM systems and their links with organizational strategies. Oiry has published many articles and chapters in books on

1 https://org-co.fr/accueil.

the uses of technology in organizations. For many years, he has been responsible for an AGHRH thematic research group on skills management.

Roxana Ologeanu-Taddei

Roxana Ologeanu-Taddei is an Information Systems research professor at TBS Business School, Toulouse, France. She is interested in the digital transformation of healthcare organizations and mHealth applications. Associate editor of the BMC Health Services Management journal, Ologeanu-Taddei is also joint head of groups concerning the digital transformation of health, firstly in the association information et management (AIM) and the association internationale de management stratégique (AIMS).

Dorsaf Omrane

Dorsaf Omrane is a lecturer in Information and Communication Sciences and joint team leader of the Organicom research team within the *Laboratoire d'études et de recherches appliquées en sciences sociales* (LERASS) of the Université de Toulouse 3 – Paul Sabatier. Her current research focuses on the content of online interactions, institutional discourses concerning the prevention and screening of breast cancer as well as perceptions and representations of actors concerned.

Hélène Romeyer

Hélène Romeyer is a professor in the Information-Communication department of Université de Bourgogne Franche-Comté, where she is director of the Information-Communication department and responsible for the Master's degree in communication. Romeyer is a researcher at CIMEOS and jointly responsible for the health, knowledge and innovations axis. Her research focuses on health in the public space: advertising, media coverage, digitization, societal movements in health (whistle-blowers, mobilizations, expert patients), and public policy changes.

Introduction

Updating Issues of Digital Health Communication

The work we present here aims to extend, develop, complete and update the various info-communication issues of digital health communication. After an overview of the challenges of the digital world on issues related to health communication, the first part of the book allows us to take a critical look at the organizational and professional limits of the field. The second part will concentrate on the links between digital health communication and a form of ethics of care. The third part will propose an overview of current issues related to the mediation of knowledge in health.

I.1. What about digital care workers?

Chapter 1, written by Benoit Cordelier, Hélène Romeyer, Laurent Morillon and Olivier Galibert, immediately allows us to illustrate the link between the deployment of DICTs in institutional medical work and the managerial constraints that aim to optimize the activities of healthcare professionals. At the heart of this desire for efficient self-standardization, the authors highlight two paradoxical injunctions produced by the implementation of the personalized medical record (PMR), considered a new tool for rationalizing management. First, this is a question of *internal mediation injunction,* which implies new forms of digital communication between professionals within the organization; these new forms sometimes come in opposition to info-communication practices that were previously institutionalized and associated with more qualitative patient care for healthcare professionals. Next, the authors identify a *disappearance injunction*, which, under the guise of efficiency, encourages the professional to use a technology whose use jeopardizes his or her

Introduction written by Benoit CORDELIER and Olivier GALIBERT.

own activity within the organization to the benefit of an improved version of the organization.

This first approach to the PMR will be continued in Chapter 2, written by Pénélope Codello, David Morquin, Ewan Oiry and Roxana Ologeanu-Taddei. The four authors propose an ambitious monographic research project on the implementation of the EMR, the electronic medical record, whose logic of digital traceability of the patient's medical characteristics, similar to the PMR, points to the same organizational paradoxes discussed in Chapter 1: the very negative feelings of healthcare professionals towards an IT tool that bureaucratizes activity and distances them from patients. Beyond the enlightening results that these researchers produce, at the crossroads of ICS and management sciences, they rehabilitate and frame the questionnaire as a valid method for studying practices. They are thus opening up new avenues of empirical investigation, by restructuring a quantitativist investigative tool that, combined with comprehensive (semi-directive interviews) and ethnographic (practice observations) tools, proves to be conducive to a form of generalization.

In Chapter 3, we will extend our investigations into new forms of technological rationalization of the production of care by moving the focus to the patients. In this research, Anne Mayère is more particularly interested in putting the patient to work through the use of digital services that aim to replace the care provided by the healthcare professional. In the already-mentioned context of reducing hospitalization time and enhancing outpatient and/or home care, telemedicine and the remote monitoring devices used imply invisible work on the part of the patient. Anne Mayère shows us how patients, remotely connected to healthcare professionals, are forced to apply protocols mechanically. They therefore undergo a form of evaluation of their performance. Taking up Foucault's concept of *pastoral power*, Anne Mayère also shows the paradox of an injunction to empower a patient who must become a co-producer of the care she or he receives, but who very often remains the executor of therapeutic processes based on a form of disciplinary power.

I.2. What about digital communication in health… ethical, empowering and emancipating?

In the second part of the book, we will focus more specifically on the digital info-communication logics likely to spread an ethic of care, synonymous with comprehensive, humanistic and emancipatory care for patients and caregivers.

In Chapter 4, the focus shifts to a more emotional approach and relational aspects of digital communication. While questioning the new mediations used between professionals for the home care of extremely vulnerable patients, Géraldine Goulinet Fité proposes revisiting the tension between cure and care through information and communication. If the cure embodies a technical medicalized approach to the individual patient, the care is part of a relational and humanistic ethics of the care of the sick person. The author relies on the observation of a socio-digital platform for coordinating the interprofessional action of the private health professionals involved in this home care. This chapter then provides an opportunity to classify SICDs with a medical aim into two main categories: on the one hand, remote monitoring techniques specific to the cure, which seem problematic in terms of their integration into care; and, on the other hand, more relational techniques, specific to care, which allow carers to express their feelings more freely about a patient's situation and which remain deeper and more valued by professionals. Taking the time to explain all of the social, psychological and emotional dimensions of the therapeutic process, Géraldine Goulinet Fité wonders whether the interactions between caregiver and patient are not to be favored in order to build a digital communication in health care that meets the ethics of care, which is accepted by all, patients and professionals alike.

Chapter 5 is an opportunity for Dorsaf Omrane and Pierre Mignot to extend this reflection on digital communication in health, which is no longer just technical, attached to the logic of the cure, but more relational, strongly marked by the ethics of care, based on remote social support. With the help of a monographic search centered on the Facebook community "*Le cancer du sein, parlons-en–!*", the two researchers point out the info-communicational limits of institutional preventive messages. In this online community for breast cancer patients, the mistrust or suspicion of persuasive messages from the community manager is revealed in the abundant interactional activity generated by messages from the patients themselves. As a result, the experiential content, valuing experience and emotion, has a greater impact. This would tend to support the hypothesis that digital communication, embodied by patients themselves and conveying all the dimensions of care, would be the most effective.

I.3. What about new digital mediations of health knowledge?

The third and last part of the book offers an overview of the changes in health expertise under the action of digital informational and communicational processes. The aim is to address, via three complementary texts, the causes and consequences of the competition between biomedical expert knowledge and lay experiential knowledge.

In Chapter 6, Hélène Romeyer therefore invites us to explore the emergence of lay medical expertise and its institutionalization in the figure of the expert patient. Based on a comprehensive empirical approach conducted through semi-directive interviews with expert patients, the reflection presented returns to the passage from a so-called paternalistic, authoritarian and top-down medicine to a so-called participatory medicine, sharing skills between health professionals and non-professionals, and supported in France by a legal arsenal that, since the Kouchner Act of 2002, encourages the patient to become a co-producer of the care he or she receives. So, how does digital communication contribute to this participatory injunction aimed at patient empowerment? Hélène Romeyer supports the hypothesis of a correlation between the professionalization of expert patients, whose role in institutions and other healthcare organizations is becoming central (notably as a vector of therapeutic education) and the mastery of digital tools. The profession of the expert patient would therefore be nourished mainly by strong skills in digital communication. From then on, the figure of the expert patient renews the issue of the patient's digital work, already addressed by Anne Mayère in Chapter 3, by insisting not on its invisibility, but on its recognition. This is not without repositioning the issues of digital literacy at the center of the reflection on the empowerment of a patient who we want to be as involved as possible in his or her healthcare journey.

Following this overview of the sociotechnical questions inherent to the figure of the expert patient, Stéphane Djahanchahi, Olivier Galibert and Benoit Cordelier propose, in Chapter 7, to continue the categorization of digital expertise in health. The aim is to understand the new mechanisms for mediating digital knowledge, which is now combined in the plural. Based on an ethnography of several online communities bringing together the actors involved in therapeutic cannabis (patients, cannabis growers, promoters of alternative medicines, etc.), the three authors update strategies for the recognition of an intra-community expertise deployed on the basis of a strong opposition with expert biomedical knowledge. Social logics of legitimization thereby emerge, produced in an info-communicational context more or less marked by an idealization of the model of the virtual or online community constituted around values of altruism, generosity and social esteem.

The last chapter of our book, Chapter 8, offers a final look at how digital mediations are being established in online health communities. Using an original semantic method for extracting conversational traces on the Doctissimo health forum, Damien De Meyere proposes an original mapping of lay expertise. For the author, lay health knowledge is divided online according to three categories of knowledge and skills acquired and shared: emotional expertise, which is acquired through interactive practices marked by empathy, interactional expertise (which sanctions users who frequently take part in more informal discussions not directly related to a pathology) and, finally, lay expertise (related to an experiential mastery of medical knowledge). While the latter form of expertise is often the most recognized and most studied, this last contribution to our overview of digital health communication shows the extent to which there is still a need for a holistic approach to online interactions. Digital health expertise must also be understood both within and beyond the realm of health knowledge. Mastering SICDs, being able to invest in interaction spaces, and being able to develop its own expression of an ethics of care are all elements that contribute to this digital lay expertise.

PART 1

Digital Patient Records: Organizational Adaptations

1

Paradoxical Changes and Injunctions in an Implementation Project of the Digital Patient Record

1.1. Introduction

Project-based change management methods rely on participation to generate support. At the same time, they multiply the activities of individuals shared between projects and operations. They place them in heterogeneous and evolving work situations, which sometimes even lead them to experience tensions in their engagement methods. The project promotes the development of complex organizational arrangements through a "myriad of locally negotiated practices and interactions" [POL 04, p. 36] that attempt to deal with what can be identified as paradoxical injunctions [MOR 09, WIT 08].

The implementation of a new tool such as the digital patient record (DPR) is an example of a project we are working on that is based mainly on document reviews and staff interviews.

The project seeks to rationalize and standardize the modalities of interaction through a specific cooperation process delimited in time. This process of cooperation implies different temporalities [COR 05], leads to disturbances in the activities of the personnel targeted by the project and generates contradictions [COR 13] to the point that some perceive a degradation of their activity and others contribute to its disappearance. For example, healthcare staff must be able to monitor patients using their records and, at the same time, let the same records go outside the health center

---

Chapter written by Benoit CORDELIER, Hélène ROMEYER, Laurent MORILLON and Olivier GALIBERT.

as part of the digitization project. These requirements, which are perceived as paradoxical, force the organization's actors to arbitrate between the project's activities and their primary activities or operations. They give rise to practices and discourses of justification that can echo individual strategies in relation to the injunctions for change, already worked on by Crozier and Friedberg [CRO 77].

1.2. Organizational paradoxes and paradoxical injunctions

The study of paradoxes and contradictions can be thought of in three strands, which, although they may be complementary and have some intersections, develop in parallel: the study of organizational paradoxes in organizational development; discursive approaches; and the mobilization, more common in information and communication sciences, of the notion of paradoxical injunction from the concept proposed by the Palo Alto school.

1.2.1. *Organizational development and paradoxes*

The trend of studying organizational paradoxes has developed more in management [HAR 17] from works such as those of [POO 89, QUI 88]. The paradox is defined there as "contradictory but [with] interdependent elements – elements that seem logical in isolation, but absurd and irrational when they appear simultaneously" [LEW 00, p. 760]. For this strand, the challenge is to find a way to reconcile contradictory elements in order to optimize the productivity of the organization [CLE 02, LEW 02, LEW 14, SMI 11]. The contradictions are integrated into the material and cultural structures of the organization [JOH 06, SMI 11]. Paradoxes are then all the more easily exercised since there is a functional interdependence that cannot be circumvented because of the speed of change or the scarcity of resources [SMI 11]. Actors cannot adapt, suffer from confusion or resist [JAR 13] until they give up and try to overcome the paradox by creating a new frame of reference [SMI 11]. For Lüscher and Lewis [LUS 08], the situation forces the actors towards a form of reflexivity that pushes them to disperse the perception of the paradox and to normalize the situation in a form of paradoxical cognition [LEW 00].

Overcoming paradoxes requires actors to be creative [QUI 88] and to put their different identities (to be understood as corresponding to their organizational affiliations) in synergy [PRA 00] in order to learn and develop [ARG 78, ARG 95]. In this way, they will be able to overcome uncertainties that block them [LUS 08]. They must then enter into a dynamic and virtuous equilibrium [SMI 11], such as double-loop learning, even if the actors may need support [VAS 17]. Behaviors that allow us to overcome are not themselves without contradictions [AND 09, AND 10,

VAS 17]. They are the result of contextual adaptations where actors use tactics to deal with the main principles or organizational lines that should be imposed on them [AND 10].

1.2.2. *Discursive approaches to the organizational paradox*

The discursive approach, also called dialectic [BEN 77, FAI 18, HAR 17], is concerned with the relationship between the discursive and material elements of the organization [PUT 15a, PUT 15b]. The originality of this perspective is that it is integrated into an approach to the constitutive communication of the organization [PUT 09].

The paradox appears in the contradiction between the practices and discourses of the organization or the entities that compose it. The contradictions are eminently social [BEN 77] and societal [SEO 02] in the sense that they are also rooted in the rhetoric that permeates society institutionally. For example, as Hargrave and Van de Ven [HAR 17] illustrate by echoing the debate between Milton Friedman and Michael Porter's views on corporate social responsibility, a particular organizational contradiction, such as the pressure exerted both to make high profits and to invest in environmental protection, is accompanied by tensions in the organization's interactions with various external stakeholders in relation to the place and role of the firm with respect to its obligations and public policies.

While the organizational development approach focuses on overcoming and on optimizing the organization, the discursive or dialectical one makes it possible to linger on the power relations between actors who confront each other through different valuations of their interests. It is therefore not so much the efficiency or productivity of the organization that is emphasized, but the rhetorical games that reflect conflicting worldviews. As interesting as organizational development approaches may be, by focusing on best practices, they oversimplify the notion of paradoxes; they neutralize it, and lead us to believe that only the convergence of actors is possible and not the crushing of one position by another, and that emotions are not an issue [PIN 19, PUT 15]. This presupposes that the individual level is taken into account.

1.2.3. *The pragmatic paradox: a return to the systemic approach of Palo Alto*

In the work of the Palo Alto school and its successors (see [WAT 79, WIN 00, WIN 01]), communication is considered a social process [LAL 15], a complex interaction that can be subject to blockages and contradictions that are difficult to overcome and therefore create distress. Non-verbal communication [BIR 70, HAL 92] may be the most obvious example of the difficulty of understanding communication that is not very explicit, or even sometimes received as contradictory. Communication is treated there as an interaction that can suffer from many modalities qualified as pathogenic. Moreover, the individual has difficulty in extracting themself from it because they do not have control over it due to the interactional nature of the exchanges. As a result, they cannot relinquish responsibility for the exchanges without breaking the relationship, which is not without negative consequences. Bateson *et al.* [BAT 56] propose the notion of a *double bind* in studies of schizophrenia to conceptualize one of the pathological modes of communication they have identified.

DOUBLE BIND. –

In a very important relationship, a speaker (1) makes an assertion (2) which they complement with an assertion about that assertion (3) so that the two are mutually exclusive. An example is “be spontaneous”. The order and the invitation to spontaneity, in other words the exercise of free will, are not compatible. Because of the paradox this creates, it is impossible for the interlocutor to conform to the message and this generates great tension, even a crisis.

METACOMMUNICATION. –

Gregory Bateson developed the notion of metacommunication to identify the corrective mechanisms of communication by drawing on cybernetic concepts where it was necessary to distinguish between information about coding elements and information about the code as a whole. Computer scientists had realized that they had to distinguish two aspects: the cues, that is, the content, and the order, that is, the relationship that will allow a command to be executed. The second level of information makes it possible to act on the understanding of the first level.

Metacommunication is therefore a communication about the set of rules in such a way that ambiguities in the interpretation of the first level communication rules can be removed.

The double binds, which are of particular interest to us, are realized when the actors are in a relationship of asymmetrical complementarity and those who are in a low position cannot obey the injunction without disobeying it. They would otherwise have to challenge the context of communication and the rules governing it, but the nature of their relationship prevents them from going outside the framework by meta-communicating without being considered insubordinate and being sanctioned.

In 1967, in the book *Pragmatics of Human Communication,* Watzlawick, Beavin and Jackson identified the characteristics of paradoxical communication. They define a paradox as a contradiction that comes at the end of a correct deduction from "consistent" premises. They then characterize three types of paradoxes: logical–mathematical paradoxes (antinomies), paradoxical definitions (semantic antinomies) and pragmatic paradoxes (paradoxical injunctions and paradoxical predictions).

Logico-mathematical paradoxes (antinomies)

Watzlawick and his colleagues define logical–mathematical paradoxes by illustrating them with Russell's paradox, which questions the idea that the set of sets not belonging to themselves would belong to itself. In a more prosaic way, this is also illustrated by the barber's paradox: a barber (a man) has the obligation to shave all men, and only those men who do not shave themselves. If he doesn't shave, he belongs to the set of people who don't (and should) shave, but as soon as he shaves, he no longer belongs to the set of people who don't shave. The absurdity of this rule cannot be overcome without moving on to a higher class or set.

Paradoxical definitions (semantic antinomies)

In fact, the contradiction can only be resolved by indicating that each set belongs to distinct *logical types*. It is therefore necessary to make it explicit with the help of specific signs that qualify the meaning of the terms. In other words, the contradiction is not so much logical as semantic since it results from a weakness in language. This can be illustrated by the paradox of Epimenides, the Cretan who would have declared: "All Cretans are liars." By not respecting the principle of non-contradiction, this sentence generates a paradox since if Epimenides is telling the truth he is lying, and if he is lying he is telling the truth. The paradox can only be solved by developing the ability to speak on language, that is, to change levels by meta-communicating.

Pragmatic paradoxes (paradoxical injunctions and paradoxical predictions)

To return to the paradox of the barber, the barber can neither act nor not act without systematically finding himself in contradiction with what is expected of him. He cannot shave or not shave without contravening the obligation. The absurd nature of this rule generates a pragmatic paradox that places the barber in an untenable position. What action to take when to obey one must disobey? The actions he could take would always be paradoxical as long as he cannot extricate himself from the communication framework in which the statement is made.

Box 1.1. *Paradoxical communication*

However, the issue at stake is not only to be analyzed at the inter-individual level. It is in the relationship between the individual and the organization that paradoxical injunctions can also appear, in the contradiction between the individual and other collective finalities [BOU 77, BOU 04, OLS 66]. The actors in an organization are often confronted with expectations that produce contradictions. The constant commitments solicited by organizations lead them to suffer the paradoxes thus generated [AUB 07, THE 04]. For Aubert *et al.* the company produces values that its employees gradually integrate. We would add that it is this mechanism that contributes to the creation of a framework, which could be qualified as ethical, that will guide their behavior and reinforce the agility of the hierarchical manager. It is interesting to note here how the passage from the individual to the collective is based on an individual effort, or rather how the passage between the micro- and macrolevels of the organization is made by submitting the individual into tension. The paradox may exist only at certain levels, but the tension preceding the effort to surpass it would essentially rest on the individual. This aspect needs to be revalued because it is, to a large extent, avoided or minimized by discursive approaches, such as those of organizational development.

1.2.4. *What divergences and convergences?*

The optimization of the organization is an important objective since its sustainability and that of its actors depends on it. However, it is not done in a blissful consensus. Actors implement circumvention or avoidance tactics. After all, contradictions, or paradoxes, are widespread in organizations. We might add that they even become normal as soon as different rationalities and purposes exist. The question is rather how they are resolved. For Bateson, Watzlawick *et al.*, the way out of the paradoxical injunction is by being able to visualize logics at different levels. This proposition is constructed from Whitehead and Russell's theory of logical types and gave rise in 1951 to the invention by Ruesch and Bateson of the notion of metacommunication, or communication about communication [BAT 95, RUE 88]. It is important to note that there is an overlapping of the levels of communication found in the second axiom of communication of the Palo Alto school (content and relation). In order to escape the paradox, we must place ourselves at the level of the relationship that includes content.

> CONTENT AND RELATIONSHIP. –
>
> Watzlawick *et al.* understand the content of the communication as the information or quantitative aspect of the communication. However, communication also relies on what Bateson calls the order of interaction. The latter is the relationship that establishes the modalities of the interaction, or behavioral injunction, which indicates the attitudes that are expected from the interlocutors. The relationship can be communicated verbally, non-verbally or based on context. It belongs to a

logical system more complex than that of content and is in itself meta-information. To explain the expectations and modalities of the relationship is to engage in meta-communication.

Josserand and Perret, whose approach can be categorized as organizational development, propose a very interesting categorization of six paradoxical organizational practices that takes into account this level issue. For these authors:

> An organization practices paradoxical management if it is able to reconcile what are usually perceived as opposing constraints. By combining constraints that are traditionally conceived as contradictory, it then enters into a virtuous circle where: "opposing values [...] remain in a state of creative tension and mutual braking. The circle is self-balancing and self-correcting" (Hampten-Turner, 1992: 36). [PER 03, p. 166]

The proposed typology is based on both:

– modes of articulation of antagonisms, which borrow the temporal logics (diachronic or synchronic) of Ford and Backoff [FOR 88];

– logics of overcoming paradoxes (differentiation, dialog, disappearance).

If the first two logics allow, for Josserand and Perret, the expression of contrary dimensions, disappearance changes the framing towards freeing the organization from the grip of the paradox.

In the case of the logics of differentiation, it is the recognition of spatio-temporal differences in the levels of analysis that makes it possible to try to think of the combination of logics not, according to the authors, in terms of exclusion, but in terms of conjunction. Perret and Josserand emphasize that there are pairs of antagonisms (micro/macro, individual/collective, etc.) and that it is the identification and recognition of these particularities of each level that allow the organization to escape the paradox. In the organization thought of in terms of process (diachronic dimension), the contradictory logics would be expressed in sequences and would exert separate influences [PER 03, POO 89, VAN 88]. With thought in terms of services and units (synchronic dimension), the two poles of the paradox would be expressed in different places and could be compartmentalized [PER 03]. Perret and Josserand propose a way out of the paradox by proposing spatio-temporal arrangements that should avoid the confrontation of contradictory logics and therefore allow the suppression of the paradoxical injunction. Let us quickly return to the definitions as proposed by Perret and Josserand of their logical category grades.

<table>
<tr><td colspan="2"></td><th colspan="3">Logic…</th></tr>
<tr><td colspan="2"></td><th>… of the differentiation</th><th>… of dialog</th><th>… of disappearance</th></tr>
<tr><th rowspan="2">Organizational practices</th><th>Diachronic dimension</th><td>Sequential practices</td><td>Stratification
Oscillation</td><td rowspan="2">Reframing</td></tr>
<tr><th>Synchronic dimension</th><td>Subdivision</td><td>Local construction</td></tr>
</table>

Table 1.1. *Paradoxical organizational logic and practices [PER 03]*

1.2.4.1. *The logic of differentiation*

Differentiation is based on Whitehead and Russell's 1910 theory of logical types and invites us to distinguish between levels of analysis. It is a reference shared with the analysis of Watzlawick *et al.* on the paradoxical injunction. However, where the latter think of the levels in terms of superposition, Perret and Josserand present them rather in terms of juxtaposition, which leads them to propose a dialog that is meant to be conjunctive rather than exclusive. However, where Watzlawick *et al.* work on a superposition of logics where one defines the rules of communication of the other, Perret and Josserand work not so much on levels of logical analysis as on levels of organizational analysis (micro–macro, individual–collective, etc.). The distinctions are relevant, but are more a matter of opposing rationalities than of paradoxes.

1.2.4.2. *The logic of dialog*

The dialog is the meeting of opposite poles in a dialectical exchange that aims at synergy or overcoming, following the example of Mary Parker Follett's notion of integration. The paradox, or contradiction, is here experienced by the actor, who finds themself at the conjunction of opposing logics. To get out of it, the dialog is either inscribed in a temporality that will lead to a stratification of practices [EVA 90] or an alternation by oscillation [BAR 79] of the imbalances brought about by the contradictions, or it plays on a specific spatiality, a local construction that facilitates arrangements impossible elsewhere. In all of these cases, it is a question of allowing the emergence of a new reality.

1.2.4.3. *The logic of disappearance*

Still, for Perret and Josserand [JOS 06, p. 173], the paradox also disappears "by a jump, the discontinuous passage from one logical level to another" because of a reframing which is above all "a displacement that frees us from the limits we apply to our cognitive field." We can return to our previous criticism of their definition of levels of logic, which seem to us to correspond more to organizational levels of analysis that may have different rationalities.

In sum, the three logics of the management of organizational paradoxes proposed by Perret and Josserand cannot be analyzed directly as resolutions of paradoxical injunctions through the metacommunication of the actors. The analytical proposals are attractive and have a certain operational efficiency, but they also have a blind spot in that they only work when the analysis is carried out on a meso- or macro-organizational level. Let us briefly return to the level of analysis and the place of the micro, or more precisely of the individual, in this model proposition.

On the analytical level, the logics as defined are rather strategies for avoiding or hiding the organizational tension created by confrontations between the logics or rationalities of the actors. Indeed, metacommunication presupposes a discussion on the rules of exchange. The raison d'être of the organizational interactions presented by Perret and Josserand remains the finality, the teleology of the organization, and not the framework of the exchange. Yet, the framework is well affected. However, this is owing to a displacement of action and its analysis. In other words, the paradoxical injunction does not disappear so much as the analyst's gaze shifts.

With regard to the place of the individual in the resolution of the paradoxical injunction, it should be stressed that most of them have a status that hardly allows them to have a strong agency on the rules that frame their actions. They do not so much discuss the reframing as undergo it.

1.3. A case study of an implementation project for digital patient records

Process improvement in health organizations is the dominant paradigm in most OECD (Organisation for Economic Co-operation and Development) countries. Reforms in the health sector are giving way to technological utopia by betting, in particular, on improved integration of information technologies. As a result, according to Kolodner [KOL 09], the model of the future is centered on the individual and on optimizing health (through prevention): it promotes self-management of health (through health support), convenience of care (through innovations such as telemedicine, telemonitoring) and coordination of care provided in multiple locations. IT is the key to making this shift successful. For the Quebec government, computerization is fully in line with this approach and is a vector for organizational rationalization and improving the productivity of the province's health network. The 2007 business plan of the *Direction des communications du ministère de la Santé et des services sociaux* (Communications Department of the Ministry of

Health and Social Services) confirms this. The regional authorities are leading the regional network computerization and electronic health record projects. Health institutions are also working to take ownership of them. The themes of rationalization, standardization, profitability of care activities and continuity of care, accessibility to information, and the choice by several advanced industrial countries of computerization and networking as a solution to the crisis in healthcare systems will probably occupy the debate for many years to come. The Quebec health record (*dossier santé du Québec*, DSQ) project is in line with these perspectives by promoting the implementation of "a tool that will make certain clinical information relevant to the monitoring and management of patients accessible electronically to authorized health professionals, regardless of where the patient receives health services throughout Quebec" (report by the *Direction des communications du MSSS*, 2007, p. 6). The electronic health record (clinical record, patient record, etc.) reveals a number of issues in the process of computerizing healthcare institutions. Among other things, this obviously affects the issue of organizational structuring and, by extension, the reorganization of the processes, professional practices and professions involved in healthcare systems.

We studied the implementation of an electronic patient record system in a health and social services center (CSSS, *centre de santé et services sociaux*). Without going into too much detail on the presentation of the field[1], we would like to return to the difficult situation experienced by certain workers whose jobs were threatened during this process of change. Archivists were in this situation. Before the new system, they were responsible for the correct classification of patient files and were in many ways important players in the reorganization of processes. As a result, they found themselves working towards the virtual disappearance of their function.

The procedure for scanning patient records involved the transfer of the records to a third party service. This meant that the records would be unavailable when they were moved. Historical records may have been unavailable for many weeks. The scanning of current records, although faster, posed other challenges in terms of processing times. Patients could return before their records were saved and made available again in the system. Also as part of this process, the individual pages of the scanned files could be returned in a jumbled fashion. These accidents, although corrected, highlighted the importance of the archivists' function both in the day-to-day running of the organization and in the more limited timeframe of the project. Prior to digitization, the archivist was the link between the various CSSS professions and branches when it came to making information available. The tasks of the archive employees were relatively varied. They were in contact with many people to ensure

1 For more details, read [COR 13].

the transmission of files. The service took on increased importance in this phase of the OACIS project. The archivists also helped to make the digitization of patient records more fluid. They ensured the proper processing of the files and even occasionally came up with new ideas to improve their functioning. However, their work becomes progressively less important as their interface function is taken over by the new system. In order to maintain a place in the organization, employees whose positions are cut are offered reassignments that are variously received and some employees have had to leave the organization. In all cases, by working on the implementation of the DPR, archivists have contributed to the disappearance of their own jobs.

The disappearance of the paradoxical injunction thus occurs here through the reassignment or the disappearance of the individual. In the first case, to return to the critical presentation of Perret and Josserand's paradox management logics, the general operating framework does not change until actors are transformed at a meso-level or disappear at an individual level.

1.4. Resolving the organizational paradox at the individual level

At the individual level, we can identify two mechanisms or injunctions that make the resolution of the organizational paradox weigh on individuals: the injunction to internal mediation and the injunction to disappearance.

1.4.1. *The injunction to internal mediation: role syncretism*

In anthropology and sociology, syncretism designates, by extension, "cases of synthesis of several cultural elements from different sources" [ANS 99, p. 515]. In the case of project-based management, this hypothesis is verified in the case of professional actors who assume, in a transitory manner, project activities. This *syncretism of roles* constitutes a contradiction imposed on the actor, which is resolved with the discontinuance of the project and produces an injunction to internal mediation [COR 06]. Actors detached from a department and involved in projects have to manage extra work and arbitrate between their obligations to their original department and those of the project team. They must therefore arbitrate on issues that are beyond their control but that they are nevertheless forced to internalize.

In the case studied, we find this injunction at all hierarchical levels, since it affects clinical managers, healthcare personnel or archivists responsible for filing patient records [COR 13]. We have insisted here on the way archivists have to deal with it, since their contributions to the effort to digitize patient records were at the intersection of their personal interests in maintaining their position and the new tasks of adaptation that the organizational change project imposed.

1.4.2. *The injunction to disappear: exit or integration*

Organizational change involves a reengineering of processes that can lead to drastic transformations, or even to the disappearance of positions or jobs in the organization. This is the case of the health center archivists here. Their contribution to the change project has the practical result of leading to the elimination of several of their positions. Their work is initially valued because they are the guarantors of the organization's memory with regard to patients. However, this memory is progressively integrated into the computerized system. They are invited to contribute to it, and this even makes up for any accidents during the digitization of archives and files in progress. The value they represent for the company is multiplied [COR 13], but does not allow them to keep their positions. The organization's recognition depends on offers of reclassification, which many refuse. The performance of archivists is then exemplary of an activity whose smooth running leads both to the disappearance of the function and the deployment of the new process. Archivists then have the choice of leaving the organization or being reclassified, which, analytically speaking, may result in the archivist being assigned to a new actor. In both cases, the archivist disappears.

1.5. Conclusion

Organizational change places pressure on the individuals who contribute to it in that the organization would like to see it resolved by those on whom it is imposed. Individuals do not always have the full capacity to do so. Matrix management, which is specific to project management, multiplies the hierarchical chains without necessarily foreseeing the methods of arbitration between logics at the intersection of which an individual, who must therefore locally manage antinomies, may find themself [COR 12]. The case of the digital patient file in a Montreal CSSS allowed us to highlight two of them: the first, the injunction of internal mediation, characterizes the fact that management modalities often ignore the contradictions to which employees are subjected and which they must resolve at the risk of mistakes; the second, the injunction to disappear, may appear rather cynical because, under the guise of organizational progress, the employee may be led to contribute to the disappearance of his or her own function.

The resolution of paradoxical injunctions occurs through a reframing that transforms the rules of operation by reengineering processes and reframing the levels of analysis more than by discussing the rules of exchange.

The doctrine of New Public Management (NPM) has been in development since the mid-1970s and the invention of the concept is attributed to Hood in 1991 in the article "A public management for all seasons", which looks at the situation in the United Kingdom. However, it was already out in the world and we find it again soon after in 1992 in the work of consultants Osborne and Gaebler. Under the influence of the Thatcher administration, the British public administration was managed with principles inherited from private business management. The latter was gaining in autonomy as well as in accountability. The principles attributed to the neoliberal movement spread to English-speaking countries, Asia and then Europe. Their reforms and public policies, the support of the World Bank and the OECD [ORG 95, ORG 05] have contributed to the diffusion of the model. The health sector is particularly targeted by these approaches (see [MCL 02, SIM 08, SIM 11]).

The NPM quickly became the bearer of an entrepreneurial vision of public administration. Although its definition varies, it is interesting to return to the trends recognized by Hood [HOO 91, p. 3] from the outset:

(i) attempts to slow or reverse the growth of the administration in terms of public expenditure and staffing;

(ii) the shift to privatization and quasi-privatization and the abandonment of core government institutions, with a renewed emphasis on "subsidiarity" in the provision of services;

(iii) the development of automation, in particular information technology, in the production and distribution of public services;

(iv) the development of a more international agenda, the issue of public management, policy design, decision-making and intergovernmental cooperation.

In the case of health organizations, rationalization on both a national and international level requires the development of computerized support for health records. This is the deployment of the electronic medical record, the computerized clinical record and even, thanks to the Internet and the growing involvement of patients themselves [HAN 18, KOL 09], of e-health records. The deployment of these information systems contributes to a management in line with NPM's policies. It aims at optimizing care processes [PAG 05, PAG 07] through a scope beyond management. Critics generally underline the detour of the consideration of the human being at the level of both employees and patients; but routinization is not always rejected, particularly among physicians who see these systems as a decision-making aid [PLU 17]. Levels of adoption are diverse. One of the paths of convergence is when healthcare professionals are able to adopt the tool to the point of integrating it into their professional identity [PET 16] and organizational culture, sometimes with a certain optimism mixed with fatalism [COR 13].

Box 1.2. *New public management and electronic patient records*

1.6. References

[AND 09] ANDRIOPOULOS C., LEWIS M.W., "Exploitation-exploration tensions and organizational ambidexterity: Managing paradoxes of innovation", *Organization Science*, vol. 20, no. 4, pp. 696–717, 2009.

[AND 10] ANDRIOPOULOS C., LEWIS M.W., "Managing innovation paradoxes: Ambidexterity lessons from leading product design companies", *Long Range Planning*, vol. 43, no. 1, pp. 104–122, 2010.

[ANS 99] ANSART P., "Syncrétisme", in AKOUN A., ANSART P. (eds), *Dictionnaire de sociologie*, Le Seuil, Paris, 1999.

[ARG 78] ARGYRIS C., SCHÖN D.A., *Apprentissage organisationnel – théorie, méthode, pratique*, De Boeck Université, Brussels, 1978.

[ARG 95] ARGYRIS C., MOINGEON B., RAMANANTSOA B., *Savoir pour agir : surmonter les obstacles à l'apprentissage organisationnel*, Inter Éditions, Paris, 1995.

[AUB 07] AUBERT N., DE GAULEJAC V., VINDRAS S., *Le coût de l'excellence*, Le Seuil, Paris, 2007.

[BAR 79] BAREL Y., *Le paradoxe et le système : essai sur le fantastique social*, Presses universitaires de Grenoble, Grenoble, 1979.

[BAT 56] BATESON G., JACKSON D.D., HALEY J. *et al.*, "Toward a theory of schizophrenia", *Behavioral Science*, vol. 1, no. 4, pp. 251–264, 1956.

[BAT 95] BATESON G., *Vers une écologie de l'esprit*, Le Seuil, Paris, 1995.

[BEN 77] BENSON J.K., "Organizations: A dialectical view", *Administrative Science Quarterly*, vol. 22, no. 1, March, 1977.

[BIR 70] BIRDWHISTELL R.L., *Kinesics and Context Essays on Body Motion Communication*, Philadelphia University of Pennsylvania Press, Philadelphia, 1970.

[BOU 77] BOUDON R., *Effets pervers et ordre social*, PUF, Paris, 1977.

[BOU 04] BOUDON R., *La place du désordre : critique des théories du changement social*, PUF, Paris, 2004.

[CLE 02] CLEGG S.R., DA CUNHA J.V., PINA E. *et al.*, "Management paradoxes: A relational view", *Human Relations*, vol. 55, no. 5, pp. 483–503, 2002.

[COR 05] CORDELIER B., "L'urgence : un outil de médiation locale dans les projets de changement organisationnel", in CARAYOL V. (ed.), *Vivre l'urgence dans les organisations*, L'Harmattan, Paris, 2005.

[COR 06] CORDELIER B., GRAMACCIA G., "Antinomies, régulations et médiations dans les projets d'innovation organisationnelle", in GERMAIN O. (ed.), *De nouvelles figures du projet en management*, EMS, Paris, 2006.

[COR 12] CORDELIER B., *Changement organisationnel et management par projet : mobilisation des systèmes d'information*, L'Harmattan, Paris, 2012.

[COR 13] CORDELIER B., "Mise en invisibilité des individus et reconnaissance des activités : un cas d'implantation du dossier patient numérique", *Communication & Organisation*, no. 44, pp. 29–40, 2013.

[EVA 90] EVANS P., DOZ Y., "The dualistic organization", in EVANS P., DOZ Y., LAURENT A. (eds), *Human Resource Management in International Firms*, Palgrave Macmillan, London, 1990.

[FAI 18] FAIRHURST G.T., "Reflections: Return paradox to the wild? Paradox interventions and their implications", *Journal of Change Management*, pp. 1–17, 2018.

[FOR 88] FORD J.D., BACKOFF R.W., "Organizational change in and out of dualities and paradox", in QUINN R.E., CAMERON K.S. (eds), *Paradox and Transformation: Toward a Theory of Change in Organization and Management*, Ballinger Publishing Company, Cambridge, 1988.

[HAL 92] HALL E.T., *Le langage silencieux*, Le Seuil, Paris, 1992.

[HAN 18] HANSEN M.M., KORNING ZETHSEN K., "Is electronic access to medical records an empowering and patient-centered initiative? – A qualitative contextual and linguistic analysis of Danish electronic records", *HERMES – Journal of Language and Communication in Business*, no. 58, pp. 157–173, 2018.

[HAR 17] HARGRAVE T.J, VAN DE VEN A.H., "Integrating dialectical and paradox perspectives on managing contradictions in organizations", *Organization Studies*, vol. 38, nos 3–4, pp. 319–339, 2017.

[HOO 91] HOOD C., "A public management for all seasons?", *Public Administration*, vol. 69, no. 1, pp. 3–19, 1991.

[JAR 13] JARZABKOWSKI P., LÊ J.K., VAN DE VEN A.H., "Responding to competing strategic demands: How organizing, belonging, and performing paradoxes coevolve", *Strategic Organization*, vol. 11, no. 3, pp. 245–280, 2013.

[JOH 06] JOHNSTON S., SELSKY J.W., "Duality and paradox: Trust and duplicity in Japanese business practice", *Organization Studies*, vol. 27, no. 2, pp. 183–205, 2006.

[LAL 15] LALLEMENT E., WINKIN Y., "Quand l'anthropologie des mondes contemporains remonte le moral de l'anthropologie de la communication", *Communiquer. Revue de communication sociale et publique*, no. 13, pp. 107–122, 2015.

[LEW 00] LEWIS M.W., "Exploring paradox: Toward a more comprehensive guide", *Academy of Management Review*, vol. 25, no. 4, pp. 760–776, 2000.

[LEW 14] LEWIS M.W., SMITH W.K., "Paradox as a metatheoretical perspective: Sharpening the focus and widening the scope", *The Journal of Applied Behavioral Science*, vol. 50, no. 2, pp. 127–149, 2014.

[LÜS 08] LÜSCHER L.S., LEWIS M.W., "Organizational change and managerial sensemaking: Working through paradox", *Academy of Management Journal*, vol. 51, no. 2, pp. 221–240, 2008.

[MCL 02] McLaughlin K., Osborne S.P., Ferlie E. *et al.*, *New Public Management: Current Trends and Future Prospects*, Routledge, London, New York, 2002.

[OLS 66] Olson M., *Logique de l'action collective*, PUF, Paris, 1966.

[ORG 95] Organisation for Economic Co-operation and Development (ed.), *Governance in Transition: Public Management Reforms in OECD Countries*, OECD, Paris, 1995.

[ORG 05] Organisation for Economic Co-operation and Development (ed.), *Modernising Government: The Way Forward*, OECD, Paris, 2005.

[OSB 92] Osborne D., Gaebler T., *Reinventing Government: How the Entrepreneurial Spirit is Transforming the Public Sector*, Addison-Wesley Publishing Company, Reading, 1992.

[PAG 05] Pagliari C., Sloan D., Gregor P. *et al.*, "What is eHealth (4): A scoping exercise to map the field", *Journal of Medical Internet Research*, vol. 7, no. 1, 2005.

[PAG 07] Pagliari C., Detmer D., Singleton P., "Potential of electronic personal health records", *BMJ*, vol. 335, no. 7615, pp. 330–333, 2007.

[PER 03] Perret V., Josserand E., *Le paradoxe : penser et gérer autrement les organisations*, Ellipses, Paris, 2003.

[PET 16] Petrakaki D., Klecun E., Cornford T., "Changes in healthcare professional work afforded by technology: The introduction of a national electronic patient record in an English hospital", *Organization*, vol. 23, no. 2, pp. 206–226, 2016.

[PIN 19] Pina e Cunha M., Putnam L.L., "Paradox theory and the paradox of success", *Strategic Organization*, vol. 17, no. 1, pp. 95–106, 2019.

[PLU 17] Plumb J.J., Hains I., Parr M.J. *et al.*, "Technology meets tradition: The perceived impact of the introduction of information and communication technology on ward rounds in the intensive care unit", *International Journal of Medical Informatics*, vol. 105, pp. 49–58, 2017.

[POO 89] Poole M.S., Van de Ven A.H., "Using paradox to build management and organization theories", *Academy of Management Review*, vol. 14, no. 4, pp. 562–578, 1989.

[PRA 00] Pratt M.G., Foreman P.O., "Classifying managerial responses to multiple organizational identities", *Academy of Management Review*, vol. 25, no. 1, pp. 18–42, 2000.

[PUT 09] Putnam L.L., Nicotera A.M., *Building Theories of Organization: The Constitutive Role of Communication*, Routledge, New York, 2009.

[PUT 15a] Putnam L.L. "Unpacking the dialectic: Alternative views on the discourse–materiality relationship", *Journal of Management Studies*, vol. 52, no. 5, pp. 706–716, 2015.

[PUT 15b] PUTNAM L.L., FAIRHURST G.T., "Revisiting 'Organizations as discursive constructions': 10 years later", *Communication Theory*, vol. 25, no. 4, pp. 375–392, 2015.

[QUI 88] QUINN R.E., CAMERON K.S., *Paradox and Transformation: Toward a Theory of Change in Organization and Management*, Ballinger Publishing Company, Cambridge, 1988.

[RUE 88] RUESCH J., BATESON G., *Communication et société*, Le Seuil, Paris, 1988.

[SEO 02] SEO M.-G., DOUGLAS CREED W.E., "Institutional contradictions, praxis, and institutional change: A dialectical perspective", *Academy of Management Review*, vol. 27, no. 2, pp. 222–247, 2002.

[SIM 08] SIMONET D., "The new public management theory and European health-care reforms", *Canadian Public Administration*, vol. 51, no. 4, pp. 617–635, 2008.

[SIM 11] SIMONET D., "The new public management theory and the reform of European health care systems: An international comparative perspective", *International Journal of Public Administration*, vol. 34, no. 12, pp. 815–826, 2011.

[SMI 11] SMITH W.K., LEWIS M.W., "Toward a theory of paradox: A dynamic equilibrium model of organizing", *Academy of Management Review*, vol. 36, no. 2, pp. 381–403, 2011.

[THE 04] THERRIAULT P.-Y., STREIT U., RHEAUME J., "Situation paradoxale dans l'organisation du travail : une menace pour la santé mentale des travailleurs", *Santé mentale au Québec*, vol. 29, no. 1, p. 173, 2004.

[VAN 88] VAN DE VEN A.H., ROGERS E.M., "Innovations and organizations: Critical perspectives", *Communication Research*, vol. 15, no. 5, pp. 632–651, 1988.

[VAS 17] VAS A., GUILMOT N., "Paradoxes et changement organisationnel : les stratégies d'adaptation des cadres intermédiaires", *Gestion 2000*, vol. 34, nos 5–6, pp. 381–410, 2017.

[WAT 79] WATZLAWICK P., BEAVIN BAVELAS J., JACKSON D.D., *Une logique de la communication*, Le Seuil, Paris, 1979.

[WIN 00] WINKIN Y., *La nouvelle communication*, Le Seuil, Paris, 2000.

[WIN 01] WINKIN Y., *Anthropologie de la communication : de la théorie au terrain*, De Boeck & Larcier, Brussels, 2001.

2

Identifying Caregiver Practices by Analyzing the Use of Electronic Medical Records

2.1. Introduction

"If I wanted to be a stenographer, I would have chosen another school!" said a pediatric surgical nurse's aide when asked about the uses she makes of the newly implemented electronic medical records (EMR) at the hospital where she works. She details:

> [The EMR] brings me irritation, annoyance, a loss of time, a loss of speed in transmissions that are so fast in writing, having to connect constantly, having to constantly change the schedules of care because they are not checked off in time and hours, in short, long live progress!

These exclamations were collected through the open-ended questions of a questionnaire on the uses of an EMR in a hospital. Addressed to all hospital clinical staff (doctors, surgeons, anesthetists, midwives), paramedical staff (nurses, orderlies, psychologists, physiotherapists), and administrative staff, this questionnaire provided information on their use of EMRs, but answer analysis also gave us very precise information on the professional practices of these employees.

Chapter written by Pénélope CODELLO, David MORQUIN, Ewan OIRY and Roxana OLOGEANU-TADDEI.

Electronic or digital medical records (EMRs) are management software that support the entire patient care process, including medical and paramedical data and reports, physician prescriptions, laboratory test results, and even room reservations and billing [XIA 12].

EMRs are supposed to facilitate medical decision-making by allowing medical information to be shared and archived across the various departments of a hospital [LAU 99, WEB 02, XIA 12]. They aim to improve the quality of care, patient safety and organizational efficiency [BAT 03]. They also aim to facilitate patient access to their medical records [ASH 07].

EMRs are thus implemented in most health organizations in numerous countries (United States [ABR 11], United Kingdom [ROB 10], Canada [PAR 14], etc.).

However, the use of EMRs by hospital clinical staff (doctors, nurses, etc.) is generally limited. Their satisfaction with this tool is generally low. They most often criticize it for being difficult to use, slow and, more fundamentally, not well suited to their professional practices. The use of EMRs by physicians and nurses is relatively low [RAH 09], as is their satisfaction. Other research [GAD 01, KHA 11, ZWA 11] identifies some perceived benefits (better electronic information exchange, access to updated information) but mostly major problems (confidentiality, security of electronic information exchange, quality of patient information, etc.).

Box 2.1. *Electronic medical record (also known as a personal digital record)*

Our chapter makes an original contribution by showing that the analysis of professional practices can be carried out using a quantitative method: the questionnaire. Generally, analyses of professional practices are based on qualitative methods, especially long ethnographic approaches. For example, [REA 13] carried out observations over six years. [NIC 11] collected data for three years. These methods allow for detailed analysis, but they are very long and do not allow the views of all staff to be collected.

Our chapter shows that, provided that conceptual and methodological precautions are taken, a questionnaire is a methodology for analyzing the professional practices of staff. Indeed, our results show that by answering questions about their use of the EMR, employees do not just talk about their use of the tool. They also detail their professional practices and the organization of their work. A questionnaire that asks questions about the uses of an EMR is therefore a methodology that makes it possible to analyze the professional practices of clinical staff.

This chapter is structured as follows. We will begin with a presentation of the existing management science literature on the uses of EMRs (section 2.2). We will then present an original conceptual framework: the "instrumental genesis" [RAB 95] (section 2.3). This is necessary to organize the analysis of the data produced by the questionnaire and to bring out results relating to the professional practices of staff. Next, we will detail our results (sections 2.4 and 2.5): we will present the professional practices revealed by our questionnaire. Finally, in our conclusion (section 2.6), we will highlight how our conceptual framework and our results contribute to the existing literature in management sciences.

2.2. Review of the management science literature on professional practices and uses of electronic patient records

There has been a "practice turn" in management science research [SCH 01]. While they had previously been largely neglected, researchers have gradually identified that professional practices are a particularly relevant starting point for analyzing organizations [BOU 90, GOM 10]. Based on a highly contextualized definition of practices [GHE 01, GHE 08], this perspective makes it possible to propose new and promising research questions. Among the questions that have already been worked on, there is the "critical role of the body and material aspects in social affairs" [NIC 10, p. 4]. In this way, this research on professional practices has been able to contribute to thinking about technological innovations in health organizations. In particular, it has shown that professional practices create social and organizational dynamics that intervene directly in the appropriation of these innovations [CRE 13].

Among the various "material aspects" that professional practice research is attempting to analyze, this chapter focuses on the electronic medical records (EMRs) that are used in hospitals.

Several studies point out that the level of use of EMRs by physicians and nurses is relatively low [EAR 09] and that the level of satisfaction of these users is also rather low. However, as seen in Box 2.1, other research [GAD 01, KHA 11, ZWA 11] identifies some perceived benefits (better electronic information exchange, access to updated information), but it mostly identifies significant problems (confidentiality, security of electronic information exchange, quality of patient information, etc.).

In their systematic review of the literature, the authors of [BOO 13, p. 15] point out that "hardware availability and system reliability, in terms of speed, availability, and freedom from failure, are necessary to ensure the use of [EMRs]." In their analytical review of the literature, [CRE 13, p. 76] confirm that the EMR:

is useful and offers relative advantages over existing practices. This is usually conceptualized in relation to speed: a new system must be at least as fast as the system that was previously operational (i.e. not significantly slow users down in their daily work).

The concept of usability is the operationalized concept that allows us to take into account the user in the design of software. This concept was designed by Nielsen [NIE 94] for human–machine interfaces. For Nielsen, usability is composed of five characteristics: being efficient, providing subjective satisfaction, being easy to learn, being easy to remember and having few errors. The pioneering work gave rise to numerous studies in ergonomics, which led to the creation of an international usability standard: the ISO 9241 standard. This standard provides requirements and recommendations for design principles and activities centered on the human operator using software during his or her work activity.

This standard is applied in the healthcare sector through several standards, including IEC 60601-1-6 and IEC 62366, which concern medical devices, the definition and certification of which are regulated by the European Union. A medical device is any instrument, apparatus, equipment, material or other article, used alone or in combination with human beings for the diagnosis, prevention, treatment of disease, injury or disability, or for the study or replacement or modification of anatomy or a physiological process.

According to these standards, usability is a measure of the effectiveness, performance and satisfaction with which specified users achieve specified objectives, in particular environments within the limits of the intended use of the medical dispositive. However, software such as the EMR is not considered as a medical device, despite the fact that it integrates drug prescribing and administration, and despite the existence of extensive literature showing that many errors in drug prescribing or administration are related to poor usability.

A variety of methods are used to evaluate and improve usability, depending on the devices lifecycle, ranging from heuristic inspection by ergonomists, according to ergonomic principles, to user tests by user profile and activity scenarios or work practices.

Box 2.2. *The concept of usability*

In this research, most of the analyses are technical [AAR 04, KUS 04, SIT 10]. They explain these weak uses and satisfactions and these difficulties through the technical characteristics of this tool.

In this chapter, we defend the idea that management tools support practices and try to make them sustainable [NIC 10] and we consider that it is possible to move towards a joint analysis of the use of tools and the transfer of professional practices.

Nevertheless, this joint analysis requires conceptual and methodological precautions to be taken.

2.3. Professional practices and the use of tools at the heart of the conceptual framework: the "instrumental genesis"

The first precautions are conceptual.

The ICS literature has gradually built the legitimacy of the concepts of tools use and appropriation. In particular, this literature has demonstrated that uses are social constructions [PRO 05]. This author identifies five currents that have, in their own way, contributed to the development of this conceptualization. Beyond Rogers' first works on the social diffusion of innovations [ROG 95], the most remarkable contributions have been those of the translation model [AKR 06], the French sociology of uses [JOU 00], ethnomethodology, the pragmatic interactionism of situated action and distributed cognition [CON 04] and the sociopolitics and critical sociology of uses [VIT 94].

We propose extending these perspectives using a conceptual framework that, while fully in line with this perspective of the social construction of uses, adds a conceptualization of work activity that is essential for us to analyze the employees' professional practices.

In this chapter, we propose to use the conceptual framework of *instrumental genesis* [RAB 95] because it has these two complementary characteristics: it is explicitly constructed to analyze the uses of the tools and it is part of the perspective of the practice [BEG 00, RAB 95, RAB 03a, RAB 03b].

INSTRUMENTAL GENESIS. –

Instrumental genesis is a theory proposed by Pierre Rabardel for reflecting on the uses of instruments [RAB 95]. This theory establishes a strong distinction between the artifact (any material and symbolic object) and the instrument, which is a social construction. An instrument is never "given"; it is constructed by the individual. It is a mixed entity, composed of the artifact, on the one hand, and the associated patterns of use, on the other hand. These usage patterns are not only individual. They have a strong collective and social dimension since their development is partly linked to interactions within the community. The process of *instrumental genesis* (the transformation of the artifact into an instrument) is structured around three dimensions. The use of the artifact questions the relationship between the individual and their activity (what he or she does, what is his or her work), to themselves (his or her identity, who he or she is) and to others (the community in which he or she works, lives, etc.).

Based on Vygostsky's perspective [VYG 34], the instrumental genesis proposes using the term *instrument* rather than *tool* in order to emphasize that an instrument does not only have technical dimensions and that it must be considered as a complex assembly of actors, actions and relationships. "Activity theory" considers that in order to analyze an activity, it is necessary to analyze the system that connects the individual, different instruments (material and conceptual), in relation to different members of the community and the objective of the activity. Adopting Leontiev's point of view [LEO 81], the instrumental genesis is particularly attentive to the collective dimension of this process [COR 13].

First of all, the instrumental genesis emphasizes that users most often faced a "system of instruments". The notion of system must be understood here in a strong sense [RAB 95]; it emphasizes that an individual never uses a single tool. The history of an organization, as well as the dynamics of the different groups of actors that make it up, means that a large number of tools have been developed [GIL 98]. [RAB 95] thus emphasizes that it is not sufficient to analyze the uses of a single tool. It is always necessary to analyze the uses of the "system of instruments", that is, all the tools that the individual uses. To analyze the uses of a given tool, it is therefore necessary to take into account the uses that it does, did or would do:

– "previous" instruments (instruments that existed before the current tool);

– "neighboring" instruments (instruments that are used in similar organizations);

– "informal" instruments (instruments that are not proposed by management but are constructed by caregivers or groups of caregivers to help them do their job and may be partly contradictory to the management imposed EMR) [GOR 95].

This is because users always compare or try to match the current instrument with these other instruments. Next, the instrumental genesis highlights the idea that the uses of an instrument systematically and simultaneously construct three types of relations [RAB 95, RAB 03b]:

– the user's relationship with their own activity (relationship with the activity);

– the relationship with others (interpersonal relationship);

– the user's relationship with oneself (reflexive relationship).

2.4. Methodology

Most research on practices is based on long periods of observation. For example, [REA 13] conducted observations for six years. [NIC 10] was present for three years. This method is particularly suitable for this type of analysis, but it is time-consuming.

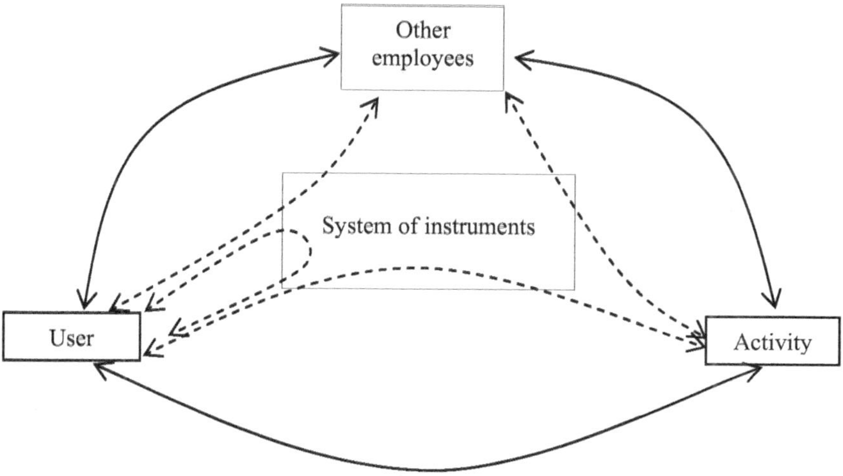

Figure 2.1. *Graphic synthesis of the conceptual framework of the instrumental genesis according to Rabardel [RAB 95]*

We used this research as the basis for our case study. We chose to collect our data in a single organization: a large French university hospital. As [NIC 10] points out, analyzing a single organization makes it possible to analyze practices within a framework of common policies and organizational principles. However, within this research, we propose enriching these analyses of practices by triangulating our data [JIC 79] and conducting a survey by questionnaire (which allows us to gather information on the practices of more than 1,000 caregivers) in addition to the interviews and participant observations.

2.4.1. *Presentation of the case*

The case study was carried out in a large French university hospital. The hospital had approximately 2,000 beds in 74 different departments. Its hospital clinical staff was composed of 900 clinicians (physicians, anesthesiologists and surgeons), 500 interns and 4,600 paramedical staff (nurses, orderlies, etc.). Each year, the hospital's activity represents an average of 235,000 stays and 540,000 consultations. Prior to the implementation of the EMR, the IT infrastructure of this hospital brought together many separate elements: electronic medical and administrative data, a system for archiving this medical data, several information systems for the different laboratories, a single storing and communication system for the different radiology departments, several specific software packages for each specialty, etc. The hospital's IT infrastructure is still very much in place today.

The EMR, developed by a software publisher is designed to support all aspects of patient care, including medical and paramedical data and reports, physician prescriptions, lab results, and even hospital bed management and billing. This EMR was implemented in nine months. The implementation led to several radical changes in the working environment of the caregivers: the disappearance of paper prescriptions, the digitalization of all the processes of care, delivery and drug inventory management and so on. The new system is now available to all caregivers, including the medical and paramedical. This implementation has led to new practices in the work, as well as in the interactions between professionals. Previously, the treatment of patients, their progress and their state of health were recorded on paper documents that were filled in by doctors, residents and other caregivers. Each department had a file for each patient that contained hospitalization records, consultation notes and test results. Every day, the treatment of patients (both inpatients and outpatients) involved accessing this file, recording and inserting new documents and using the information stored in it.

By the end of EMR implementation, all departments (except for resuscitation) had digitized the drug process from prescription to delivery with more than 1 million lines of prescriptions per year. The results of both biology and imaging tests of all patients were included in the EMR. Paramedic transmissions, prescriptions and patient discharge letters were integrated into the EMR in a paperless environment. However, physicians were free either to put their medical notes in the EMR or to leave them on paper only. This means that, two years after the end of the implementation, some departments no longer use paper, while others keep paper records.

The objective of our study was to identify practices related to the use of EMRs. We chose to analyze the uses of all types of hospital staff (doctors, surgeons, anesthetists, nurses, nurse managers, midwives, medical secretaries, physiotherapists, dieticians, psychologists, etc.). We administered our questionnaire 21 months after the end of the implementation of the EMR. This deadline had not been decided at the beginning of the project. It was set according to the priorities of the hospital management, which considered that the questionnaire should be administered several months after the implementation of the EMR.

2.4.2. *Data collection and analysis methods*

One of the authors of this chapter is a doctor in this hospital. He is responsible for the *Délégation pour l'information hospitalière* (DIH), which aims to promote the safe use of EMRs and adapting its configuration to the work of hospital clinical staff. Among his various activities, this author organized a committee for structuring the EMR to allow decision making by the various professional groups on the necessary changes. The objective of this committee was to carry out a continuous analysis of the uses of the EMR and to modify its parameters in order to develop and facilitate these uses. For the purposes of this research, this author is therefore part of a "reflexive" research approach.

Another of the authors of this chapter is a researcher who has completed over 450 hours of non-participant observation in 18 months (between September 2014 and February 2016), in particular in meetings of this committee. During this observation, the author also conducted informal conversations before and after the meetings with the participants of the meetings, held informal conversations with the physician members of this committee, conducted seven semi-directive interviews with the hospital management, kept 2,835 emails received and collected internal reports and the minutes of each of these meetings. Observation data and interviews were transcribed in full. All of these data were coded. The codes used were mainly taken from the literature (practices, uses, appropriations, etc.) and the conceptual framework used (relationship with oneself, relationship with others, relationship with the activity). However, some codes emerged from the data themselves (such as the question of the governance of the organization or the collective good).

In collecting these data, these two authors have developed a real familiarity with the field, professional practices and uses of EMRs.

In addition, in order to understand the perceptions of clinical staff with respect to EMRs, a questionnaire was developed and administered by these two authors. This questionnaire included closed-ended questions (e.g. about the features of the EMR used by the respondent), but in this chapter, we analyze only the open-ended questions at the end of the questionnaire. These included: "From your point of view, what are the benefits of EMR (called EMR-X)?" and "From your point of view, what problems do you have with EMR (called EMR-X)?"

Our methodological objective here was data triangulation [DEN 78]. We gathered different kinds of data (observations, interviews, documentation and questionnaires) on a single subject in order to better understand it [JIC 79].

The objective of this triangulation was to seek a convergence of results on a given phenomenon in order to reinforce the validity of our study and to intentionally confront situations where the results were different in order to highlight the different perceptions and uses among caregivers. These similarities and differences allowed us to formulate new interpretations of the phenomenon we were studying and thus produce new knowledge [GRE 89].

We collected 1,292 completed questionnaires (for a population of 6,443 caregivers). Details are given in Table 2.1.

We coded the answers to the questionnaire using the concepts of instrumental genesis [RAB 95]. For example, some of our codes were: relationship with activity; relationship with oneself; and the system of instruments. We added new codes that emerged from the analysis of the responses themselves. For example, we added new codes for the different instruments that were used (such as "museum" or "source") or for the technical dimensions of uses (such as "ergonomics").

Professions	Population	Responses to the questionnaire	Response rate
Healthcare assistants	1,740	78	4.48%
Anesthesiologists	131	28	21.37%
Social workers	59	45	76.27%
Nurse executives	250	56	22.40%
Surgeons	172	35	20.35%
Dentists	71	5	7.04%
Nurses	2,014	426	21.15%
Residents (medicine or surgery)	280	52	18.57%
Interns (pharmacy)	20	4	20.00%
Physiotherapists	145	30	20.69%
Doctors	844	171	20.26%
Pharmacists	71	20	28.17%
Midwives	99	18	18.18%
Medical secretaries	547	151	27.61%

Table 2.1. *Population and questionnaire responses*

2.5. Results

By analyzing the answers to the questionnaire, we found many opinions on the technical difficulties encountered in the use of this instrument. Nevertheless, we propose going beyond them to analyze how these answers give us information on the relationship to the activity, to others and to oneself.

2.5.1. *Technical dimension of uses*

In the answers to the open-ended questions on the questionnaire, we find the classical themes of the technical analysis of the tools.

Users found that this tool made it easier for them to find patient information, reports, and to access the information they needed. For example, one physician (a pediatric intern) pointed out that EMR-X allowed “easy retrieval of patient history.” A geriatric nurse’s aide pointed out that with EMR-X she “doesn’t have to go upstairs to look for patient records.” An anesthesiologist pointed out that “the advantage of the prescription software is that, for nurses, the prescriptions are clear: no illegible handwriting or 1cp x 2 (without knowing the duration or dosage of the drug).”

On the other hand, many of the comments were less positive. Here too, it is possible to make a predominantly technical analysis. For example, users very frequently mentioned the technical problems they encountered when using the software. For example, this caregiver said:

> The connection is too long. You have to click twice on your ID, which wastes time. Then, the records are not in alphabetical order and it’s complicated to change the dates.

An orderly stated:

> There is also a big issue at night when there is an “update” of EMR-X because then we can’t access it for several hours.

She even backed up her statement with precise details: “(e.g. Wednesday 08/01/2014 from 4:00 to 6:30 am)”, while a nurse wrote:

> Software unsuitable for my workplace; too slow; frequent bugs; messy windows where nothing jumps out.

Another nurse (in surgery): “BUGS, BUGS, BUGS, that’s all I remember!!!!!!”

Criticisms of ergonomics were also less general and based on specific elements of the activity. For example, an anesthesiologist explained: “In prescriptions, it is very complicated to give information in open field for nurses: be careful with one thing or another…”

Similarly, one nurse stated, “there has been no training adapted to the particularities of the service,” and many mentioned the lack of training in the use of this EMR. Even when training had taken place, it was considered insufficient. As one nurse stated: “In fact, the EMRX training lasted 30 minutes, which explains my dissatisfaction with its use.”

It would therefore be quite possible to make a purely technical analysis of these uses and their difficulties. However, the analysis of these uses seems to us to be enriched if we go further. It seems relevant to us to consider it the starting point of the analysis and not the end of it. The conceptual framework of instrumental genesis allows us to carry out such an analysis [RAB 95].

2.5.2. *System of instruments*

When we go beyond the analysis of the technical dimensions of the instruments, we find in the answers to the questionnaire the mention of a very large number of instruments other than the EMR-X that we questioned the users about. If we look at the different categories proposed by the instrumental genesis, we see that the respondents' answers constantly evoke several elements.

First, "previous" instruments are instruments that existed before the current tool. Many people spoke of "Musée", a tool that existed before the current one. For example, a psychiatrist explained:

> I don't see why, for example, we have to rewrite the patient's name in full, when it would be so much smarter to have a patient list to check off, as we used to do in MUSEE.

Given the strong criticisms of EMR-X, these references to previous tools often point out that they were more adapted to the professional practices of these personnel.

Secondly, "neighboring" instruments are instruments used in similar organizations. An anesthesiologist says:

> You don't even have to talk about it, it sucks! Just look at the software used at T. (NDA: EMRs used in a hospital 30 km away) to see that you can do much better. It's not one or two improvements that are needed, it's everything that's wrong!

Many of them also compared with the tools they used in their private life (or even in certain professional activities). One midwife described it this way:

> In the age of tablets and smartphones, the use of EMR-X is not at all intuitive. Many steps must be performed before arriving at the information you are looking for or writing down information.

Others made comparisons with the paper records that existed or still exist. For example, one caregiver stated:

> There is a large loss of transmissions, diets not transcribed on our schedules because it takes longer to log on to EMR-X than it does to open our old binders to check a diet or a prescription.

Others compared this tool to the information that some experienced colleagues could give them. For example, a psychiatric nurse said, "Some of my colleagues answer my questions when I can't find information."

Finally, "informal" instruments are instruments that are not proposed by management but are constructed by caregivers (or groups of caregivers) to help them do their job and may partly contradict the EMR imposed by the management [GOR 95]. For example, one nurse stated: "At the moment we use 'Source' for our patients, which I find much more appropriate and more confidential." Similarly, dentists continue to use a tool other than EMR-X.

2.5.3. *Relationship with activity, with oneself and with others in the use of EMRs*

The conceptual framework of the instrumental genesis allows us to enrich this analysis of the system of instruments by emphasizing that uses fall within three different relationships: with the activity, with oneself and with others.

2.5.3.1. *Relationship with activity*

The answers to the questionnaire are, first of all, striking in the number of respondents who described their activity to show that their work was specific and different from that of their colleagues, that the EMR failed to take into account the specificity of their activity and, in doing so, did not really succeed in supporting them in carrying it out.

A health nurse manager in surgery said:

> We urgently need more visible planning that includes the patient's name, the physician in charge, the care to be provided, the tests to be done and the pathology. Caregivers need this holistic view of their patients in care so they can be responsive and not have to go patient by patient.

In the same way, a midwife said:

> As a midwife many things are not suited to our profession. Being both prescribers and executors, we have to do things twice (prescribing to ourselves, and ticking off the care once it has been done) and this generally takes more time than it did previously with paper records. We have not followed the training for doctors (prescribers) and so many of us do not always master all the functionalities.

We could find comments in each of the professions for which we have respondents.

In fact, one of the conclusions that can be drawn from this analysis is that the EMR is built on the pattern of an adult patient, in general medicine and for a short hospital stay. For all other configurations, the EMR is not suitable [OLO 15]. This configuration is certainly the most common in a hospital of this type. However, the sum of the other "specific" configurations (children's hospitalization, obstetrics, long or recurrent hospitalizations, etc.) is much higher [OLO 15] in number than this "dominant" configuration. This means that there are far more cases where the technology scripts listed in this EMR do not correspond to the day-to-day practices of professionals.

The EMR, which promotes a cross-functional perspective of healthcare organizations, comes up against an organization that is still very strongly characterized by a high degree of specialization by function and by department. The promotion that the EMR is attempting to make of the transversal perspective is explained by the desire to rationalize the economy of healthcare organizations, as well as by the objectives of improving the speed and quality of the information sharing in this type of organization.

Analysis of the questionnaire responses clearly shows this tension between the scripts in the EMR and employees' practices. By answering about their use of the EMR, they then provide us with precise information about what their activity is.

2.5.3.2. *Relationship with oneself*

In talking about their activity, respondents also spoke about themselves, and how they saw themselves and their professional identity.

For example, the responses to this questionnaire included responses that could not have been found in any other type of organization. Many professionals justified their criticism of the EMR by the risk of prescription error, for instance. A physician in pediatrics explained this as follows:

> If the nurse makes a mistake in entering the weight (there have been several times a one-line discrepancy with a temperature entered in the

> weight box, making big differences with an infant), there is a risk of error because the software directly calculates the prescription in mg/kg. There is then a high risk of overdose....

A surgical nurse manager was also concerned that EMR-X does not alert us to inconsistencies in prescribing and prescribing a treatment to which the patient is allergic is always possible.

Other professionals clearly indicated in their responses how they saw their role in the hospital. One female doctor said: "A resident in surgery is not meant to push a cart!"

As is customary in identity dynamics research, we are led to identify differences between groups. A pediatric resident thus clearly stated:

> There should not be the same interface for doctors and nurses. Things may appear clearly or prescribed for the doctor, but not for the nurse where everything is mixed up in terms of care.

Another doctor did not share this opinion since he criticized the tool by saying: "Why are there differences between what the doctor prescribes and what is readable into the EMR: why is the visual not the same????"

This also led to stating the professional evolutions which are not accepted. A nurse's aide declared: "We don't have the time to take care of our patients in their entirety because the computer has become the priority to our great despair!"

These responses make it clear that the uses of EMR fail to contribute to the realization of the professional identity of these professionals and the professional practices that would be necessary to achieve this.

2.5.3.3. *Relationship with others*

Talking about their activity and who they were, employees also talked about their relationships with others, that is, how they saw them and how they worked (or didn't work) with them.

More critical statements reflected, for example, the conflicts that existed between professional groups. A surgical intern castigated "the 'sacrosanct' nurse's reply: not prescribed, not done, which leads to delays in care".

[RAB 15] has shown that this is always the case, that is, he use of the tool reveals the relationship with the activity, with oneself and with others.

However, this is probably even truer in the case of health organizations. Patient care involves different professions (different medical specialties, nurses, healthcare managers, medical secretaries) who must coordinate and share information. Care is an interdisciplinary process that is in tension with the functional bureaucracy that the hospital represents. As a complex professional bureaucracy [BOO 14], the hospital is characterized by divergent goals [GLO 01] and multiple stakeholders [BOO 09]. All employees, because of their expertise and personal efficiency, must specialize in one activity (surgery, radiology, occupational therapy, etc.), but the patient is cross-functional in relation to all these activities: the same person is operated on, X-rayed, cared for by the occupational therapist, etc. [BOO 10]. In a way, the patient "compels" the employees of the different professions to work together.

If we take up the midwife's comments above, we may form the impression that each employee's activity is so different that it is impossible to have a common tool (such as the EMR). However, it is made indispensable because the patient is cross-functional to the activity of all of these employees and they must therefore transmit information about the care that has been provided to a particular patient from one professional specialty to another. These transmissions require a common tool even if it sometimes seems impossible to make it exist.

It is also significant that the most positive employees with respect to the EMR are the secretaries, in other words, one of the professional groups that is explicitly dedicated to the coordination between the different professionals. A secretary in pediatrics stated:

> [EMR-X] gives me information about patients, allows me to type their email, bill the consultations and output the requested results.

Another stated:

> The patient record is visible in its entirety. […] The recording of reports is made easier thanks to the database of doctors' addresses. There is also a follow-up on the "status" of the reports (to be edited, signed, sent, etc.).

2.5.4. *Debates on the common good*

The analysis of the answers to the open-ended questions in this questionnaire on the uses of the EMR does not only inform us about the relationship of its users to themselves, to others and to their activity. We also find traces of real debates on what constitutes the "common good" in a healthcare organization.

For example, most caregivers would agree with the physician's statement: "Basically, we want to give our patients the best, but I don't feel that this tool really helps us achieve that goal…."

Another doctor (in dentistry) explained:

> We all feel like we spend more time with the computer than we do with the patient. What a paradox for a (hospital) care center!!!!! In the end, the time spent is not spent with the patient: a very bad experience for a caregiver!

A doctor hid his disappointment behind humor:

> Thanks [name of EMR designer], lean management and other marketing bullshit: to make successful software, you have to start from the ground up and create it with the people involved on a daily basis. I hope this supplier doesn't work on Airbus because seeing "restart Xnet" mid-flight is a blow to not knowing if you have enough kerosene to get home….

Another physician linked the EMR to the financial dimensions that are increasingly present in care and care organizations. Noting that the instrument did not meet his professional needs, he made an assumption: "We had to take the cheapest one, as usual."

A psychiatric nurse even lent intentions to those who designed this tool, as well as to those who conceived the questionnaire (and by extension to the entire hospital management?). When asked about the benefits of EMR-X, he answered: "None and your questionnaire is unhelpful… The sentences are perverse… As perverse as your EMR-X is."

2.6. Conclusion

These results make it possible to develop three avenues for discussion with the existing literature.

First, this research shows that the use of an EMR that has just been implemented in a university hospital is a particularly interesting time to gather information on the practices, knowledge and work of caregivers. The post-implementation phase is a specific moment when nothing is yet "taken for granted" and everything can be questioned. New practices are not yet institutionalized [REA 13]. More often than not, the implementation of EMRs destabilizes pre-existing practices. It can even destroy some of these particularly crucial practices and greatly reduce the effectiveness of healthcare teams. By trying to explain what is destabilized by the implementation of EMRs, caregivers verbalize practices that could, until now, have been almost unconscious and thus allow us to analyze them.

Second, using the conceptual framework of instrumental genesis [RAB 95], this research shows that the analysis of the uses of an EMR is not only technical, but also gives us precise information on the relationships that users have with their activity, themselves and others. The analysis of the responses shows that users make numerous criticisms about ergonomics, technical connection difficulties and so on [RAB 95]. Even if they exist, these criticisms of the technical dimension of the instrument are often linked to the user's activity. As a result, these remarks cannot be considered purely technical. They also express the user's relationship with his activity. For example, many responses detail how the activity is remote and different from the implicit case of an "adult patient in general practice and short hospital stay" that was used to construct this EMR. In doing so, most often, these caregivers develop a reflexivity about themselves ("a surgical resident is not meant to push a cart!") and about others ("the 'sacrosanct' nurse's reply: not prescribed, not done, which leads to delays in care").

In addition to this, we came up against some particularly stimulating reflections on the transmissions that are really necessary between these employees and on the instruments that could improve them: one EMR, several EMRs, a modular EMR? With all of these remarks, we have a complete and detailed reflection on what a university hospital is. What are its strategic objectives? How are the different professionals supposed to work and collaborate in this organization?

Third, the results of this research have methodological implications. It uses a questionnaire to identify practices. This is an unusual method for this type of topic. Ethnography is most often used because practices are highly contextualized. Our results show that we arrive at an identification of practices that is much less precise than that which can be obtained through ethnography [NIC 10]. However, it allows us to have a much more general view of the practices in this hospital. This was possible because:

– our questionnaire concerns the uses of a tool that is supposed to affect the activity of employees directly;

– we use a conceptual framework that is in line with the practice-based perspective. With this type of conceptual framework, we are able to distance ourselves from the technical discourse on tools;

– our questionnaire was distributed in a post-implementation phase (practices had not yet really been institutionalized [REA 13]). After this phase, institutional work will have been done: it will have led either to the rejection of the tool or to its appropriation, but, in any case, the discourse on practices would have been much more difficult to identify;

– we did not rely only on a questionnaire. We triangulated our data [JIC 79] with participant observation, non-participant observation, interviews and, finally, a questionnaire;

– we analyzed the open-ended questions in these questionnaires. These two questions dealt with the benefits and problems of this EMR. Their analysis shows that it is probably futile to seek further refinement in the formulation of these questions. Indeed, on many occasions, we found that even in the question on the benefits of the tool, employees responded on its limitations. It seems to us that this error cannot be corrected by greater refinement of the questions. These respondents are so filled with anger about this tool slowing them down or preventing them from doing their job that, even when asked about the benefits, they see only the limitations. For example, a female epileptology doctor answers the question about the benefits of EMRs: "NONE, and to make sure you read it, I'm putting it in twice!" and she reproduces the same critical text in the question about the benefits and in the question about the problems.

The results obtained in this research show that a questionnaire makes it possible to analyze the professional practices of personnel in health organizations.

These results appear to be fully valid in the case study we conducted. However, their external validity will need to be reinforced by further research in other organizational contexts and using other tools.

However, these results already make it possible to consider a particularly stimulating line of research: the detailed analysis of the role of instruments in professional practices in healthcare organizations. Indeed, instruments appear to be much more important in the transformation of practices than the literature generally suggests.

2.7. References

[AAR 04] AARTS J., DOOREWAARD H., BERG M., "Understanding implementation: The case of a computerized physician order entry system in a large Dutch university medical center", *Journal of the American Medical Informatics Association*, vol. 11, no. 3, pp. 207–216, 2004.

[ABR 12] ABRAMSON E.L., MCGINNIS S., EDWARDS A. *et al.*, "Electronic health record adoption and health information exchange among hospitals in New York State", *Journal of Evaluation in Clinical Practice*, vol. 18, no. 6, pp. 1156–1162, 2012.

[AKR 06] AKRICH M., CALLON M., LATOUR B., *Sociologie de la traduction. Textes fondateurs*, Presses de l'École des Mines, Paris, 2006.

[ASH 04] ASH J.S., BERG M., COIERA E., "Some unintended consequences of information technology in health care: The nature of patient care information system-related errors", *Journal of the American Medical Informatics Association*, vol. 11, no. 2, pp. 104–112, 2004.

[BAT 03] BATES D.W., EBELL M., GOTLIEB E. *et al.*, "A proposal for electronic medical records in US primary care", *Journal of the American Medical Informatics Association*, vol. 10, no. 1, pp. 1–10, 2003.

[BEG 00] BEGUIN P., RABARDEL P., "Designing for instrument-mediated activity", *Scandinavian Journal of Information Systems*, vol. 12, no. 1, pp. 173–190, 2000.

[BOO 09] BOONSTRA A., GOVERS M.J., "Understanding ERP system implementation in a hospital by analysing stakeholders", *New Technology, Work and Employment*, vol. 24, no. 2, pp. 177–193, 2009.

[BOO 14] BOONSTRA A., VERSLUIS A., VOS J.F., "Implementing electronic health records in hospitals: A systematic literature review", *BMC Health Services Research*, vol. 14, no. 1, p. 1, 2014.

[BOU 90] BOURDIEU P., *The Logic of Practice*, Polity Press, Cambridge, 1990.

[CON 04] CONEIN B., "Cognition distribuée, groupe social et technologie cognitive", *Réseaux*, vol. 22, no. 124, pp. 53–79, 2004.

[COR 13] CORDELIER B., "Mise en invisibilité des individus et reconnaissance des activités : un cas d'implantation du dossier patient numérique", *Communication & Organisation*, vol. 44, no. 1, pp. 29–40, 2013.

[CRE 13] CRESSWELL K., SHEIKH A., "Organizational issues in the implementation and adoption of health information technology innovations: An interpretative review", *International Journal of Medical Informatics*, vol. 82, no. 5, pp. e73–e86, 2013.

[DEN 78] DENZIN N.K., *The Research Act*, 2nd edition, McGraw-Hill, New York, 1978.

[GAD 01] GADD C.S., PENROD L.E., "Assessing physician attitudes regarding use of an outpatient EMR: A longitudinal, multi-practice study", *Proceedings of the American Medical Informatics Association Symposium*, p. 194, 2001.

[GHE 01] GHERARDI S., "From organizational learning to practice-based knowing", *Human Relations*, vol. 54, no. 1, pp. 131–139, 2001.

[GHE 08] GHERARDI S., "Aujourd'hui les plaques sont molles !", *Revue d'anthropologie des connaissances*, vol. 2, no. 1, pp. 3–35, 2008.

[GIL 98] GILBERT P., *L'instrumentation de gestion – la technologie de gestion, science humaine*, Economica, Paris, 1998.

[GLO 01] GLOUBERMAN S., MINTZBERG H., "Managing the care of health and the cure of disease – Part I: Differentiation", *Health Care Management Review*, vol. 26, no. 1, pp. 56–69, 2001.

[GOM 10] GOMEZ M.L., "A Bourdieusian perspective on strategizing", *Cambridge Handbook of Strategy as Practice*, pp. 141–154, 2010.

[GRE 89] GREENE J.C., CARACELLI V.J., GRAHAM W.F., "Toward a conceptual framework for mixed-methods evaluation designs", *Educational Evaluation and Policy Analysis*, vol. 11, no. 3, pp. 255–274, 1989.

[JIC 79] JICK T.D., "Mixing qualitative and quantitative methods: Triangulation in action", *Administrative Science Quarterly*, vol. 24, no. 4, pp. 602–611, 1979.

[KHA 11] KHAJOUEI R., WIERENGA P., HASMAN A. *et al.*, "Clinicians satisfaction with CPOE ease of use and effect on clinicians' workflow, efficiency and medication safety", *International Journal of Medical Informatics*, vol. 80, no. 5, pp. 297–309, 2011.

[LAU 99] LAU F., DOZE S., VINCENT D. *et al.*, "Patterns of improvisation for evidence-based practice in clinical settings", *Information Technology & People*, vol. 12, no. 3, pp. 287–303, 1999.

[LEO 81] LEONTIEV A.N., *Problems of the Development of Mind*, Progress, Moscow, 1981.

[MCG 11] MCGINN C.A., GRENIER S., DUPLANTIE J. *et al.*, "Comparison of user groups' perspectives of barriers and facilitators to implementing electronic health records: A systematic review", *BMC Medicine*, vol. 9, no. 1, p. 1, 2011.

[NIC 10] NICOLINI D., "Practice as the site of knowing: Insights from the field of telemedicine", *Organization Science*, vol. 22, no. 3, pp. 602–620, 2010.

[NIC 12] NICOLINI D., *Practice Theory, Work and Organization. An Introduction*, Oxford University Press, Oxford, 2012.

[NIE 94] NIELSEN J., *Usability Engineering*, Elsevier, Amsterdam, 1994.

[OLO 15] OLOGEANU-TADDEI R., GAUCHE K., MORQUIN D. *et al.*, "The appropriation capacity: A neglected intangible organizational capacity in the adoption of information and management systems", *Innovations*, no. 2, pp. 79–100, 2015.

[PAR 14] PARÉ G., RAYMOND L., DE GUINEA A.O. *et al.*, "Barriers to organizational adoption of EMR systems in family physician practices: A mixed-methods study in Canada", *International Journal of Medical Informatics*, vol. 83, no. 8, pp. 548–558, 2014.

[PRO 05] PROULX S., "Penser les usages des TIC aujourd'hui : enjeux, modèles, tendances", in VIEIRA L., PINED E. (eds), *Enjeux et usages des TIC : aspects sociaux et culturels*, vol. 1, pp. 7–20, Presses universitaires de Bordeaux, Bordeaux, 2005.

[RAB 95] RABARDEL P., *Les hommes et les technologies, approche cognitive des instruments contemporains*, Armand Colin, Paris, 1995.

[RAB 03a] RABARDEL P., WAERN Y., "From artefact to instrument", *Interacting with Computers*, vol. 15, no. 5, pp. 642–645, 2003.

[RAB 03b] RABARDEL P., BOURMAUD G., "From computer to instrument system: A. developmental perspective", *Interacting with Computers*, vol. 15, no. 5, pp. 665–691, 2003.

[RAH 09] RAHIMI B., TIMPKA T., VIMARLUND V. *et al.*, "Organization-wide adoption of computerized provider order entry systems: A study based on diffusion of innovations theory", *BMC Medical Informatics and Decision Making*, vol. 9, no. 1, p. 52, 2009.

[REA 13] REAY T., CHREIM S., GOLDEN-BIDDLE K. *et al.*, "Transforming new ideas into practice: An activity based perspective on the institutionalization of practices", *Journal of Management Studies*, vol. 50, no. 6, pp. 963–990, 2013.

[ROB 10] ROBERTSON A., CRESSWELL K., TAKIAN A. *et al.*, "Implementation and adoption of nationwide electronic health records in secondary care in England: Qualitative analysis of interim results from a prospective national evaluation", *BMJ*, vol. 341, p. c4564, 2010.

[ROG 95] ROGERS E.M., *Diffusion of Innovations*, 4th edition, Free Press, New York, 1995.

[SCH 01] SCHATZKI T.R., "Introduction: Practice theory", in SCHATZKI, T.R., KNORR-CETINA K., VON SAVIGNY E. (eds), *The Practice Turn in Contemporary Theory*, Routledge, London, 2001.

[SIT 10] SITTIG D.F., SINGH H., "A new sociotechnical model for studying health information technology in complex adaptive healthcare systems", *Quality and Safety in Health Care*, vol. 19, no. 3, pp. i68–i74, 2010.

[VIT 94] VITALIS A., *Médias et nouvelles technologies. Pour une sociopolitique des usages*, Apogée, Rennes, 1994.

[VYG 78] VYGOTSKY L., *Mind in Society*, Harvard University Press, Cambridge, 1978.

[WEB 02] WEBSTER A., "Innovative health technologies and the social: Redefining health, medicine and the body", *Current Sociology*, vol. 50, no. 3, pp. 443–457, 2002.

[XIA 12] XIAO N., SHARMAN R., SINGH R. *et al.*, "'Meaningful use' of ambulatory EMR: Does it improve the quality and efficiency of health care?", *Health Policy and Technology*, vol. 1, no. 1, pp. 28–34, 2012.

[ZWA 11] ZWAANSWIJK M., VERHEIJ R.A., WIESMAN F.J. *et al.*, "Benefits and problems of electronic information exchange as perceived by health care professionals: An interview study", *BMC Health Services Research*, vol. 11, no. 1, p. 1, 2011.

3

Communication Approach to Patients' Health Work: Remote Relationship and Intertwined Powers

3.1. Introduction

The general context of health and the healthcare system in France is characterized by an aging population as a whole (and an aging medical population in particular), the increase in social inequalities in health and the rise in the number of patients with chronic diseases. These changes are felt all the more as policies aimed at controlling public budgets dedicated to healthcare institutions, combined with professional logics, have led to a concentration of the most specialized healthcare institutions and professionals in metropolitan areas, with the result that access to care is difficult in what are referred to as "medical deserts". Finally, the offer of care in healthcare institutions remains structured in "silos" by pathology, as does most of the training of future practitioners [CHE 15].

In recent decades, and particularly since the 2000s, public health policies have promoted an "outpatient shift", primarily to contain the costs of the healthcare system. This orientation is reflected in the priority given to "first resort" medicine (general practitioners) and day hospitalization, and in the reduction of medium and long stays. The evolution still in progress is now showing its full effects, which are paradoxical in some cases[1]. The healthcare system has "turned the corner", and the

---

Chapter written by Anne MAYÈRE.

1 As a result, it appears that the number of medical acts carried out by general practitioners has decreased since 2005, and that patients are making greater use of hospital consultations, owing to the decrease in the number of general practitioners and the reduction in their working

resulting acceleration raises questions about the changes as they manifest themselves, what they do to patients and caregivers and what the latter do with them.

The prioritized orientations aim to promote the development of outpatient care and everything that facilitates the maintenance or return home of patients. However, these patients are increasingly suffering from chronic diseases, often presenting several pathologies. This results in treatments with associated effects that can be disabling and that vary according to the patient and the period of time. These long-term treatments require strict compliance with medical instructions and a capacity to detect and react to symptoms, that is, renewed forms of self-care and self-monitoring[2] [GUI 15]. The aim is to avoid a "loss of opportunity"[3] in configurations where the caregivers themselves cannot provide care or check the progress of patients, as is the case in medium or long-stay hospitalization. They effectively meet patients only during consultations or outpatient hospitalization, knowing that everything is being done to ensure that these moments are spaced out over time and that they are densified and optimized[4].

In such a context, the question of patients' work is being raised in a new way. New dispositives are being deployed in the field of e-health with the argument of improving care and access to care. How do they fit into the work and with patients? In what way do they contribute to renewed forms of rationalization extended to the work of patients through the improvement of disciplines [HEL 05]?

---

hours. This trend is expected to increase since "in 2013, 49.5% of GPs were over 55 years old (compared to 11% in 2000)" [BRA 16, p. 76].

2 Studies show that one in two patients with chronic diseases no longer comply with drug prescriptions, or go so far from the dosage that it is ineffective, after one year of treatment.

3 Loss of opportunity is a notion specific to the field of law and litigation, defined by the *Cour de cassation* as "the current and certain disappearance of a favorable contingency" (Cass. 1re civ. November 21, 2006, no. 05-15-674). The loss of chance includes both the deprivation of a future gain and the occurrence of a risk that could have been avoided. It is an injury that can be invoked by any victim in the context of a dispute over administrative or judicial liability, whether in tort or in contract. The compensation awarded by the judges does not correspond to the damage linked to the lost gain or to the deleterious consequences of the risk that has arisen, but is measured after an evaluation of the extent of the lost opportunity, by awarding a fraction of this damage (Cass. 1re civ. July 16, 1998, no. 96-15.380).

4 Medical consultations are indeed governed by a set of obligations and protocols. It is appropriate for practitioners during a consultation to carry out several activities in a combined manner, such as conducting an investigation, examining or consulting test results, informing, obtaining the patient's informed consent, issuing a prescription, therapeutic education, etc., all within a time frame under budgetary and queue management constraints.

To examine this evolution, we will start with the notion of "patients' work" [COR 85, STR 97]. Initially, this notion was developed by health sociologists to account for the fact that, even in hospital settings, patients had to co-produce care. These researchers have shown that this work is invisible, and that its non-execution or partial execution can be sanctioned by moral judgments, or even by differentiated forms of treatment. Patients are thus led to conform to what is expected of them, to be "patients" and "good" patients.

MEDICAL DESERT. –

The notion of "medical deserts" refers to the unequal distribution of health professionals and, more broadly, of the supply of care in a territory. This issue became a major focus of public debate in France at the end of the 1990s, through the positions taken by elected officials and those, varying in time and content, of the Order of Physicians and practitioners' unions. It was taken into account and relayed by the media following the dissemination of demographic projections, and was thus established as a public health problem [DEP 15]. The criteria suggested for identifying under-endowed areas are mainly the distance to be traveled for treatment and the time required to make an appointment. In 2015, 27% of French people said they had difficulty getting an appointment with a general practitioner within a reasonable time, and 55% said they had difficulty getting an appointment with a specialist (BVA survey cited by [BRA 16]). The debate first concerned what is referred to as "city medicine" or "primary care" as opposed to hospital, that is, general practitioners, private specialists and private nurses. This debate gradually extended to healthcare institutions, as hospital centers or specialized hospital services (such as maternity wards) were closed. While "medical deserts" primarily concern rural areas far from the metropolises, the question of accessibility to care now also extends to metropolitan areas. Indeed, access to so-called "first resort" care, primarily GPs, is becoming more difficult with the retirement of practitioners (in 2013, 49.5% of GPs were over 55 years old), with the development of their lifestyles towards greater control over their working hours, while the overall population is aging and is increasingly affected by chronic diseases. Moreover, incentives aimed at a better distribution of GPs across the territory have not had a significant effect. What is referred to as the "crisis in emergency services" is thus attributed to this difficulty in accessing care; 60–70% of emergency room visits concern patients who could not be treated elsewhere because they had no access to a doctor (*Le Monde*, June 14, 2019).

3.2. Reconstructing patients' work

The work of patients was largely ignored in the conception of a patient as the "object of care", with acute diseases and care during hospitalization as the primary reference points. This is now taken for granted in the predominantly outpatient-based healthcare system, without being recognized as such. The reorganization of healthcare institutions as "care factories" [PIE 11], in *lean management* with optimized inventories and lead times, presupposes that each patient lends himself or herself to being both an efficient object of care and a subject able to practice home care and its follow-up.

Patients must be autonomous and efficient, they have responsibilities to fulfill, they are recipients of care and they must comply with the constraints and expectations associated with it.

This evolution of the user–client–consumer required as a co-producer is characteristic of contemporary societies and extends to a wide variety of products and services, particularly health services [DUJ 08]. We will see how the notion of "autonomy" is invested to justify transformations aimed at ensuring that patients – presented in certain discourses that claim to be disruptive and modern as "clients" – contribute effectively to the process of "care". This new figure of a self-care provider and patient–partner reflects "the shift from a homogenizing form of health government (government through social) to an individualizing form (remote government)" according to "new biopolitical control strategies typical of neoliberal societies" [NOU 10, p. 327], emphasizing the autonomy and responsibility required of patients.

Patients' work is increasingly carried out at a distance from the caregivers, without the caregivers being able to exercise direct control. This concerns a growing part of what conditions patient survival and the control of the disease. This is why dispositives have been developed to monitor patients remotely. We will use the notion of "pastoral power", formulated by Foucault, to characterize what is at work in the caregiver–patient relationships thus reconstructed [MAR 10]. We will see how the configurations of distance care lead to reliance on pastoral power to ensure that patients conform to the discipline required by the medical responsibility delegated to them, through the implementation of a relationship to self and to illness as prescribed by medical knowledge [GUI 15]. In this maze of interlocutors and organizations, and in the face of the accumulation of tasks and skills required, some patients get lost or silently give up, for lack of resources and support, precisely because they are vulnerable because of their illness, or because they refuse these interwoven forms of power extended to their daily lives.

OUTPATIENT SHIFT. –

The so-called "outpatient shift" is an overall orientation of public policies related to the health system. Initiated in the 1990s in some Western countries, it has underpinned public health policies in France since the 2000s. According to this position, the aim is to entrust "primary care", local or "first resort" professionals – primarily referring physicians – for piloting and taking charge of patients' "health pathways". This means refocusing the intervention of healthcare establishments on the most specialized technical procedures, limiting the length of hospitalization and thus of costs. In particular, "day hospitalization" is being promoted, with the development of "outpatient surgery" being highlighted as emblematic and a model to be systematized. Such a development presupposes that primary care is accessible, which is not necessarily the case (see the definition of medical deserts in section 3.1). The need for renewed cooperation between professionals, based on so-called ambulatory structures (health centers, territorial health communities), as well as the sharing of information through the shared medical record (EPR), is also emphasized. However, such prerequisites have been stated for a long time without having been put into practice. While "meeting patients' needs" is considered central, the question remains open as to what this "outpatient shift" does to patients and their families, particularly in the French context, which is characterized by strong social inequalities in health.

3.2.1. *Recomposed and multiplied patients' work*

3.2.1.1. *Patient work: a concept linked to very topical issues*

The concept of patients' work is intended to reflect what patients are expected to do. Strauss *et al.* have identified three dimensions of patient work [COR 85]:

– work directly related to the illness, such as making appointments, attending examinations, complying with instructions, taking medication according to the prescribed dosage, etc.;

– work on daily life with the disease, which relates to the various prescriptions for it, such as a particular diet, recommendations for physical exercise and everything involved in carrying out these daily activities with the effects of the disease;

– emotional work, which consists of facing the biographical rupture induced by the announcement of the disease, anguish in the face of this disease and the various social judgments made about the patients. Indeed, especially in the case of chronic diseases, prejudices tend to designate these patients as being primarily responsible for their illnesses.

Strauss showed that these three dimensions of work are closely interrelated and interact, with a change in one of them having implications for the others.

Chronic illnesses, long on the margins of the healthcare organization model, have gradually become a fact of society, owing to medical progress and longer life expectancy. In order to cope with these developments, various hospital laws have aimed to reorganize institutions and the healthcare system in general. As a result, the

HPST law (2009 law on hospital reform and patients, health and territories) plans to "link the territory" through healthcare institutions, territorial groups and strengthened links between local hospitals and university hospitals.

Medicine has long expected patients to be "compliant", obediently submitting to tests and treatments. Since the 1950s, associations of patients with chronic diseases have been trying to promote the need for practitioners and public authorities to take into account the conditions of living with the disease. From the 1980s onwards, patients and patient associations demanded the recognition of specific knowledge and an active role for patients [BAR 05].

The notion of empowerment finds one of its main origins in a contestation of power and domination, as identified at the micro-social level in doctor–patient relationships, and at the macro-social level in what is referred to as a medical elite linked to political powers and potentially under the influence of the pharmaceutical industry. A completely different origin is that of consumer movements that claim extensive access to information to enable informed choices, and access to the most innovative treatments via practitioners selected and compared iteratively according to objective criteria [BAT 12].

The law of March 4, 2002 on patients' rights and the quality of the healthcare system enshrined the patient's right to be informed of his or her state of health and the principle of free and informed consent; "health democracy" requires that users be represented in the various bodies of healthcare institutions.

However, has the power of the patient become, above all, the power of the market [BAT 12]? The rationalization of health organizations (generalization of managerial methods, etc.) is a major challenge. According to some authors, the industrialization of services, creating the conditions for interchangeability between doctors and encouraging them to favor standards over singularity, would go hand in hand with the emancipation of patients. Codified relations would hinder the possibility of dialog and deliberation, with "choices" being constrained by opposable medical references and protocols, medico-legal obligations and economic requirements. The "right to health" would have become a "duty to health", with individuals subject to self-governance techniques, equipped with surveillance technologies [NOU 10]. Furthermore, the "autonomous", "responsible" patient, in charge of his or her "self-management", in "self-care", referred to in discourses promoting empowerment, is conceived in a decontextualized, desocialized way, which, by the same token, can contribute to reinforcing social inequalities in health, owing to all that is postulated in terms of dispositions, support and resources. Patients would in fact be confronted with what remains to be done, remains to be said, remains to be understood, remains to be coordinated and remains to be paid in an outpatient-based care system that limits situations of interaction.

Box 3.1. *Empowerment, health democracy and health*

In addition, and following the movements of patients' associations (particularly those of patients affected by HIV) and various scandals in the health sector, patients' rights have evolved, particularly with the law of March 4, 2002, on patients' rights and the quality of the health system. This new legislative framework states that patients must be informed and must participate in therapeutic decisions in order to give informed consent [CAR 14].

At the convergence of these developments, which were very quickly and therefore briefly sketched out, a profound transformation in the patients' work took place. Without this work being designated as such, it is required and extended more than ever, in the course of the recompositions associated with the ambulatory organization of care. The "patient" must be autonomous; regularly referred to as "at the center of the health system", he or she is supposed to be equipped with new empowerment.

To understand what is at work in this promotion of autonomy and empowerment in health, we will draw on some key contributions from Marie-Anne Dujarier's research exploring the work of the consumer. To question the way this work is equipped, conformed and controlled, we will use the notions of pastoral power as worked out from Foucault [HEL 05, MAR 10, NOU 10].

3.2.1.2. *Consumer work extended to health services*

Speaking of the consumer's work, Marie-Anne Dujarier reminds us that "work is a social relationship, a socialized and socializing activity" [DUJ 08, p. 15]. "Then, and to differentiate it from leisure, work creates value for the company: it is an economic criterion. Finally, we speak of work as an activity of the subject in touch with reality and constraint, struggling with it to try to develop his material, social and subjective environment." [DUJ 08, p. 15] As Dujarier specifies, "to work is to put one's heart into it" [DUJ 08, p. 16].

The consumer's work has two dimensions: productive work, on the one hand, and organizational work, on the other hand. The second refers to "all collective activities that contribute to making an organization, [...] to name and relieve the multiple contradictions that run through the activity" [DUJ 08, p. 16]. After the contradictions unresolved by the governing bodies and intermediate hierarchies have been transferred to the most operational employees [DEG 05, DEJ 13], it is more and more consumers or users who have to deal with them. Consequently, they have to implement a great deal of organizational work in order to find acceptable forms of resolution. In addition, tasks and costs are outsourced, which they have to take on (for instance, concerning products, final assembly or technical tests according to instructions transmitted remotely, etc.).

This consumer work is increasingly equipped. The technologies thus implemented present different facets from the point of view of work: "they can be prescriptive when they frame the operator's activity" [DUJ 14, p. 31]; "they can have an operational function when they carry out a task"; and "finally, the technologies can participate in the control of the activity and the measurement, in real time, of its productivity" [DUJ 14, p. 31]. For example, in healthcare, patients are equipped with "PRO – Patient-Reported Outcomes" applications, which are applications through which they must record their health status in standard formats. Their work is framed by an "architext" [JEA 99] that specifies the questions, the authorized answers and their sequences. This work is controlled and "scored" through the measurement of punctuality and regularity; patients who are not very "observant" are then called upon to question these "omissions", which generate alerts and reduce the system's performance indicators.

The arguments that are used refer to improved monitoring, as well as to an organizational need to respond to the growing number of users. As Dujarier points out: "following the example of participative management used with employees, the "motivational" discourse addressed to the consumer then plays on the arguments of autonomy in the activity" with three associated arguments: "you win"; it is "for your comfort and safety"; and a third argument, often prevalent in commercial offers, equivalent to "you have no choice". The registers are thus intermingled, suggesting an increased autonomy, which is in fact a constrained autonomy, that of directed self-production, even if it means "softening it by adding a suggestion of a relationship during the performance" [DUJ 08, p. 83].

Dujarier questions a "more experienced than observed autonomy" in that this possible feeling is accompanied by an "increased dependence on organizations" [DUJ 08, p. 201]. It is therefore important to question what would be a "paradoxical injunction to constrained autonomy", with the norm of being autonomous becoming "a moral burden" [DUJ 08, p. 202]. For Dujarier, "the increase in the feeling of autonomy, quite different from the gain in real autonomy, is a denial of our fundamental heteronomy" [DUJ 08, p. 202]. Indeed, this evolution, much more than *personalization*, goes in the direction of *individualization*, assuming that consumers/users select in standard formats what is the least distant from their own situation.

As in any social relationship and, moreover, in any work relationship, a power relationship is at work. It is appropriate to explore what these power relationships are in the recomposed caregiver–patient relationship. To do so, we will use the notions of "pastoral power" and "disciplinary power" to question the relationships in remote patient monitoring.

3.2.2. *Relationship of care and intertwined "pastoral and disciplinary powers"*

In contemporary societies, a new productivity is expected from individuals through the valorization of "positive figures of health, virtue and happiness" [MAR 10, p. 26]. Renewed social norms relating to the governance of bodies are being established through diffuse forms of power that participate in the government of the self and others [MAR 10]. Normative judgment and scrutiny are among the techniques through which this power is operationalized by "seeking to give individuals self-discipline and control over their own person" [MAR 10, p. 28].

Questioning more specifically what is at work in care relationships, Martin proposes exploring the issue of "pastoral power":

> Pastoral power is a form of power that allows one person (a "guide") to influence the subjectivity of another through control and dependence, causing the latter to become attached to their own identity through a mechanism of awareness of their personal knowledge. [MAR 10, p. 28]

This power is present in relationships involving some form of "caring for the other". We hypothesize that this pastoral power is reconfigured when care is provided on an outpatient basis and remotely, with each patient being invited to tell the truth about himself or herself in a telephone dialog combining distance and a reconfigured form of intimacy. Control, which cannot operate through direct constraints on the body and on the source of activities, is delegated to the instruments and to the patients in the form of self-control.

Pastoral power is equipped with various techniques, particularly "confessional techniques", through which the individual is encouraged to "go even further in his private revelations" [MAR 10, p. 29].

The effectiveness of such a process relies on the fact that "the appropriate individual must be persuaded that this is not an interrogation but a therapeutic process that is carried out under the aegis of an ethical principle of non-maleficence" [MAR 10, p. 29].

Pastoral power is not unidirectional; it is exercised over the various parties involved in the exchanges, because "everything that is governed must, in fact, be governed" [MAR 10, p. 32]. As a result, caregivers are both instigators and objects of this power, which governs their approach to patients and their relationships with patients. In particular, reflexive practice, which has long been taught to nurses and which is now explicitly required of practitioners, can be considered as mobilizing self-technologies aimed at controlling these ways of doing and thinking in order to verify their compliance with “best practices”, as specified by academic knowledge.

In section 3.3, we will specify the field of study and the method used before further investigating, on the basis of this theoretical support, how remote relationships come to reform patients’ work, and what they give to see on the powers thereby equipped.

3.3. Field and method

The dispositive under study is presented as providing non-medical home monitoring for patients with heart failure. The study presented here was a clinical trial, designed according to the standard model of evidence-based medicine. It was a randomized controlled trial involving more than 990 patients. The patients were divided into two groups by a random draw, with one group of patients each equipped for 12 months and one group of non-equipped patients monitored according to the standard of care. Since the Social Security Financing Act of 2014, new modes of funding have been authorized for approved remote monitoring devices, on the basis of a flat rate per patient treated. In line with the “Prospective e-Health” report drawn up under the auspices of the Ministry of the Economy in 2016, which states that solvable demand is not on the side of patients, the experiment aims to convince public funders of the benefits of this remote monitoring. The “social and organizational acceptability” study, an ancillary study carried out in addition to the main study, aimed to identify the success factors and potential sources of blockages or obstacles. The aim was to characterize the conditions for successful enrolment (as defined in [LAT 92]), or the potential reasons for failure, for patients and those who contribute to their care, and for the health professionals directly concerned [BEN 17][5,6].

In the system studied, a private company is the operator of the study and employs the staff of the remote monitoring center, which consists of a secretariat, a technical service in charge of sending materials and a team of nurses. Three items are sent to each patient: a scale with a digital display and a start button (battery

5 This research program benefited from the financial support of the University Hospital of Toulouse and of the LABEX SMS (ANR-11-LABX-0066). M. Bénéjean and then K. Swiderek acted as project leader researchers, with the participation of E. Coeurdevey in the research field work, and contributions from I. Bazet, E. Fournalès, P. Marrast, N. Haschar-Noé and T. Lang.

6 The entire study, including the acceptability study, received the agreement of the *Comité de protection des personnes* – Committee for the Protection of Persons – and of the CNIL – Commission Nationale de l’Informatique et des Libertés.

operated); a box that must be connected to the electrical network at all times and positioned near the scale; a folder dedicated to therapeutic education. The remote monitoring system includes a daily collection of clinical data consisting of the measurement of the patient's weight and her or his answers to eight questions related to the pathology (and its symptoms) through the use of a box.

Algorithms analyzing this data generate alerts in the event of missing measurements or data exceeding pre-established thresholds, alerts that are transmitted to the nurses at the monitoring center. A telephone call is then required within 24 working hours to validate the clinical reality of the symptoms and encourage the patient to consult his or her attending physician in the event of an alert[7]. In addition, the service is based on a "structured telephone follow-up": after the first calls to establish the basis of the follow-up relationship, scheduled appointments follow, approximately every three weeks, dedicated to the therapeutic education of the patient.

The corpus of our study is composed of 47 in-depth semi-directed interviews, conducted for between 1.5 and 2.5 hours, with patients equipped at their home. The sample is not random but significant [KAU 11], in order to account for the variety of patients in terms of sex, age, location and other socio-demographic characteristics. Particular attention was paid to issues of inequalities in health and access to care, including patients living far from urban centers, as well as patients from diverse professions and socio-professional categories, including those who are or have been farmers, employees, workers, artisans and shopkeepers. We also made sure to meet both men and women.

In addition, 10 interviews were conducted with staff members of the remote monitoring center, and 22 interviews were conducted with healthcare professionals working with these patients (including 13 attending physicians). The analysis of the material is based on a thematic analysis, relying in particular on the identification of intriguing episodes, repetitions and contradictions, in a grounded research approach based on a back-and-forth with progressively refined readings [CHA 06].

3.4. Remote relationship and intertwined powers

We will further explore the results of this analysis to characterize the relationships that take shape with such a remote monitoring dispositive, exploring what putting patients to work involves pastoral power, disciplines and dispositions.

---

7 Advice of the *Commission nationale d'évaluation des dispositifs médicaux et des technologies de santé* (National Commission for the Evaluation of Medical Devices and Health Technologies), September 6, 2016 (p. 5).

3.4.1. *Establishing the relationship and learning to talk about oneself*

3.4.1.1. *Building proximity remotely*

Research on remote medicine dispositives emphasizes the significant change for nurses in not being in physical proximity to the patient. Physical proximity is important in usual care practice in that it supports narrative proximity, and gives caregivers a sense of an overview of the patient and his or her situation [MAL 03]. It provides a variety of indications on skin tone, posture, gestures and walking, as well as smells and touch (heat, moisture, skin consistency), knowing that these proximity-based skills are developed more specifically during training and in the practice of the profession. Physical contact, beyond care, is "an invitation to reunite or re-anchor the patient in a liveable relationship with his or her body" [MAL 03, p. 2317]. Moreover, physical proximity and face-to-face relationships allow for diversified non-verbal expression, supportive gestures and so on. For nurses working in patients' homes, support in understanding the situation is taken from the home environment, its layout, its upkeep, those who live there and those who visit it.

Nurses from the remote monitoring center "visit" the patients at their homes via the telephone. The sense of hearing is therefore the first to be required, as other research also shows [OUD 11]. The staff at the remote monitoring center develop active listening skills, paying attention to weak signals and to all auditory clues that can be picked up from the tone of voice, rhythm, breath, noise or the absence of ambient noise. Exchanges with family and friends, when available, and possibly with caregivers visiting patients at home, in some cases, allow the nurses at the remote monitoring center to access cues from a delegated physical proximity, and to give meaning to remote measurements or signals.

What our interviews reveal is how, during this experiment, the nurses from the remote monitoring center worked a lot to build such narrative and moral proximities with the patients. For many patients, this work is in large part, if not essentially, the basis for their adherence to the dispositive as a whole. In a way, the disciplinary power associated with the dispositive itself (weighing oneself, answering questions, keeping telephone appointments and the associated rules) and with the lifestyles it aims to promote, and what pastoral power requires in terms of self-revelation, seem to be justified and counterbalanced, for many of the patients we met, by the relationship as perceived with the nurses. It should be noted that these patients, who are often elderly, find that their opportunities for social interaction are reduced by their illness. For many of these patients, the quality of the relationship thus established with the nurses is what makes it possible to overcome certain elements of the system that irritate or exasperate them, from the box and its synthetic "voice" to the statements of therapeutic education.

3.4.1.2. *The call as a technology of self-revelation*

To make remote monitoring effective, the nurses try to build up proximity remotely and to gradually get the patients to talk of themselves, and to talk about their work directly related to the disease (taking medication, examinations, etc.) and about daily life with the disease (respect for a low-salt diet, adapted physical exercise, etc.). It is on the basis of all the information gleaned, the "confessions" obtained during the calls, that the nurses orient their remarks and, in particular, the themes of future calls. This in-depth knowledge is also used when they receive alert messages following the automated treatments operated by the algorithms[8], to determine the action to be taken, taking into account the estimated effectiveness of the alert.

Pastoral power is thus equipped with self-revelation technologies aimed at patient expression in accordance with the expected contribution. The form of attachment built up over the course of the calls also aims to ensure the effective availability of patients, who must be close to their (wired) telephone and available during telephone appointments.

This relational construction is based on a form of affective work, which consists of creating proximity and attachment remotely. At the same time, nurses must conform to an authorized discourse within the limits of their area of authority. The operators of pastoral power are thus governed both by texts delimiting their field of intervention and by the algorithms that trace their actions and that they must inform. Part of the know-how deployed seems to consist of ensuring that patients adhere to the dispositive, through a form of individualization of the approach and discourse, while complying with the prescribed discourse.

For patients who are tired from their illness, often elderly ones, accepting phone calls is not a matter of course, especially since they are a personal target of telephone marketing and have often been alerted to the associated risks. The familiarity built into the relationship encourages them to accept a third party, an "absent other" [GID 84], in the manner of a host, in a civil relationship that compensates for the potential intrusion of these telephone calls and the questions asked. The establishment of this familiarity is all the more necessary since the questions addressed concern daily life with dimensions relating to intimacy and to the patient's body. These questions lead to elements of family and social life being addressed, and assume that he or she lends himself or herself to self-auscultation and reporting. It is therefore important that the questioning is not perceived as an interrogation but as a voluntary expression.

---

8 Based on weight measurements and responses to questions from patients, these algorithms identify discrepancies or combinations of responses to questions that may indicate risks of cardiac decompensation.

3.4.1.3. *An enabling power relationship in a context of loss of control*

Any power relationship is both enabling and constraining in various ways [GID 84]. In this case, patients report an exchange distinct from outpatient visits, which allows them to revisit episodes that are precisely so dense and constraining that they do not find any help to give meaning to what happens to them. As a result, with the remote monitoring nurses, the form of the exchange and its regularity can make it possible to address questions that cannot be raised during the constrained appointments with specialists. These interlocutors are also appreciated in that they try to make the information intelligible and adapt it to the patient's situation:

> Patient: It did help me a lot. And then I have questions, because the problem is that the doctors they put the bit between your teeth and then it's "we are registering you on the waiting list, your heart has this, this, this and this." Well, okay, and they give loads of information and you have to try to remember everything. So I don't retain half of it, and then, once they've said their stuff, there are questions, but at the time, the questions don't come to me. And then you leave because all you want to do is go home and that's it. So it's good to have someone where I know that if I have a question to ask, she'll be able to answer me and then that's it; in terms of the transplant, how will it be afterwards, the time it takes....

This ability to reformulate, explain and unfold the undertones and explicit medical speech also derives its effectiveness from the fact that it takes shape over time, with regular appointments that allow patients and distant nurses to follow up on a question, to return to an aspect that is misunderstood or reconsidered, or to prepare for a near future that is still partly unknown. Outpatient care in fact divides the care pathway into highly specialized micro-episodes whose overall meaning patients are trying to grasp, and in which they try to construct a role for themselves as subjects.

3.4.2. *Intertwined disciplines*

3.4.2.1. *The discipline of the sociotechnical dispositive*

The remote monitoring dispositive involves inserting activities related to remote monitoring into daily life, which is already under great strain owing to illness: weighing oneself as much as possible at a fixed time, and then answering the box's questions and making oneself available for telephone appointments. This work is considered very limited by the practitioners promoting the dispositive: "three minutes a day". When tested in practice, it appears that the design of the device, even in its most trivial materiality, includes assumptions concerning the patients and their lives: for example, elderly patients who are not supposed to be mobile (there is no provision for simple portability of the device) and who live according to very regular schedules [MAY 18]. However, it appears that even elderly patients vary in their schedules, precisely in changing activity, place to keep the taste for life.

3.4.2.2. *The discipline of daily life: the "low-salt" diet*

A "low-salt" diet is part of the usual daily living prescriptions for patients with cardiovascular disease. For some patients, telephone calls are a beacon to maintaining alertness:

> Patient: I know at least that I'm "under surveillance", in theory, and that, anyway, it's up to me to be careful, or with my wife to be careful with what I eat, etc., etc. So, it suits me very well.

Even if patients may find it necessary to set up their own framework to make these prescriptions acceptable:

> Researcher: Have you attended any therapeutic education sessions?
>
> Patient: Careful, we're going to get into some nasty stuff here. If you talk to me about nutrition, I'm not talking anymore! [...] I have a holy horror of nutritionists. [...] They're people who pretend to deliver the holy word [...]. I listen to my priest when I'm interested. When he doesn't interest me, I don't listen to him!

By expressing himself in this way, this patient evokes how pastoral power can be the instrument or the entry point of a disciplinary power, and he shows how previous social learning is used to refuse or appropriate such a dispositive.

This is one of the tensions to which follow-up nurses must respond: they are supposed to limit themselves to the precise script of the referenced and authorized speech, given that they do not have medical authority. At the same time, they must ensure that patients adhere to the dispositive which requires forms of individualization that adjust the standard recommendations to the patient's situation as identified during exchanges and as measured by the instruments.

3.4.2.3. *Allowing oneself a lack of discipline*

Some patients allow themselves to insert their tempo, to put the dispositive on hold by leaving the scenario thus constructed, even if it means checking its safety with the doctors they happen to meet as part of the follow-up of their disease. One patient explained to us how she allowed herself to "go on strike". The expression used is quite meaningful when it comes to a dispositive that is supposed to help patients, but which turns out to require additional work, with the patients being trapped in the experience of the disease:

> Patient: So, I went on strike for eight days, it pissed me off. [...] Then I said to myself, I'm fed up, I will not weigh myself for a while and here I am... And I ignored the scales.

A not insignificant number of patients enrolled in the experiment returned the technical device before the end of the 18-month period, the staff in charge of the experiment having negotiated with a few others so that they no longer had to respond while keeping them in the experiment.

3.5. Conclusion

With the evolution of a healthcare system that prioritizes outpatient care, patients are seeing their work grow and transform. They are asked to be "actors" in their own health, "autonomous" and "responsible". Much of the work they have to do takes place outside of healthcare establishments. It involves increasingly demanding and complex activities, such as taking new molecular therapies including targeted therapies based on specific dosages, monitoring of test results and treating drug-related effects that can be very debilitating. For this work, patients are informed and often trained according to the behavioral standards advocated by the "therapeutic education of the patient". They must keep their records up to date in a context where, more than ever, integration is manual; the continuity of patient records is built manually, on foot, the patients bringing the required elements with them. In the most advanced work configurations, patients can be equipped with PROs or "patient- reported outcomes", a name that evokes the operator of industrial processes. This work equipment is often combined with telephone follow-ups, according to various economic and organizational configurations.

Based on an in-depth case study, we have questioned what happens in the relationships thus equipped and distributed, how they are established, invested and maintained – or not. We have highlighted how such relationships mobilize renewed pastoral power in configurations where patients are encouraged, remotely, to monitor themselves according to medical standards. This pastoral power, like any power, is variously empowering and constraining; some patients have told us that they have learned to speak and listen to certain signs from their bodies that they had previously ignored. Pastoral power is intertwined with disciplinary power, itself recomposed with what is required by the discipline of the sociotechnical dispositive, combined with the discipline of work directly related to the illness and of the work of daily life with the illness. Patients must comply with detailed instructions, as close as possible to their daily lives, and ensure their traceability.

What is argued and potentially perceived as a support is based on work, the relationship representing a key component of this work, with its techniques and tools. Patients speak to us directly or indirectly about this work and these working relationships, evoking their assiduity and their seriousness, as well as their escapes, or even their "strike". This work presupposes dispositions, largely hidden by a universalizing promotional discourse.

Dujarier showed how much the "autonomy" increasingly invoked could be constrained. The associated forms of rationalization of relationships are forms of individualization, not personalization, with an associated denial of our fundamental heteronymy [DUJ 08]. It is appropriate to question these rationalized and equipped forms of patient work and relationships, including the risks that they may entail. In the most commercial configurations, it may turn out that sick people only have access to circumscribed, priced, standardized relationships. In other configurations, the transformations under way may reinforce the invisibility of relational work of personalization, at the risk of exhausting the caregivers who feel they have to ensure it.

3.6. Acknowledgments

I thank Éléonore Coeurdevey, Pierre Delcambre, Elisabeth Fournales, Nadine Haschar-Noé and Thomas Heller for their proofreading and all their suggestions, while retaining full responsibility for the limits of this writing.

3.7. References

[BAR 05] BARBOT J., "How to build an 'active' patient? The work of AIDS associations in France", *Social Science & Medicine*, no. 62, pp. 538–551, 2005.

[BAT 12] BATIFOULIER P., "Le marché de la santé et la reconstruction de l'interaction patient-médecin", *Revue française de socio-économie*, no. 10, pp. 155–174, 2012.

[BEN 17] BENEJEAN M., MAYERE A., "Ordres de temporalité et médiations dans le travail de santé : le cas de patients dotés d'un équipement de télémedecine", in LAMY A., CARRÉ D. (eds), *Temporalités et dispositifs de médiation*, L'Harmattan, Paris, 2017.

[BRA 16] BRAS P.-L., "Les français moins soignés par leurs généralistes : un virage ambulatoire incantatoire ?", *Les Tribunes de la santé, Presses de Sciences Po*, no. 50, pp. 67–91, 2016.

[CAR 14] CARDIN H., "La loi du 4 mars 2002 dite 'Loi Kouchner'", *Les Tribunes de la santé, Presses de Sciences Po*, no. 42, pp. 27–33, 2014.

[CHA 06] CHARMAZ K., *Constructing Grounded Theory, A Practical Guide Through Qualitative Analysis*, Sage Publications, Thousand Oaks, 2006.

[CHE 15] CHEVREUL K., BRIGHAM K.B., DURAND-ZALESKI I. *et al.*, "France. Health system review", *Health Systems in Transition*, vol. 17, no. 3, 2015.

[COR 85] CORBIN J., STRAUSS A., "Managing chronic illness at home: Three lines of work", *Qualitative Sociology*, vol. 8, no. 3, pp. 224–247, 1985.

[DEG 05] DE GAULEJAC V., *La société malade de la gestion, idéologie gestionnaire, pouvoir managérial, et harcèlement social*, La Découverte, Paris, 2005.

[DEJ 13] DEJOURS C., "Effets de la désorganisation des collectifs sur le lien… À la tâche et à l'organisation", *ERES, Revue de psychothérapie psychanalytique de groupe*, vol. 2, no. 61, pp. 11–18, 2013.

[DEP 15] DEPLAUDE M.-O., *La hantise du nombre, une histoire du numérus clausus de médecine*, Les Belles Lettres, Paris, 2015.

[DUJ 08] DUJARIER M.-A., *Le travail du consommateur, De MacDo à eBay : comment nous coproduisons ce que nous achetons*, La Découverte, Paris, 2008.

[GID 84] GIDDENS A., *Les conséquences de la modernité*, L'Harmattan, Paris, 1984.

[GUI 15] GUIRIMAND N., "De la 'pédagogisation' des soins des malades chroniques aux dispositifs d'éducation thérapeutique", *Le Télémaque*, no. 47, pp. 59–70, 2015.

[HEL 05] HELLER T., "De l'anatomopolitique à la psychopolitique", *Études de Communication*, no. 28, p. 13, 2005.

[JEA 99] JEANNEREY Y., SOUCHIER D., "Pour une poétique de 'l'écrit d'écran'", *Xoana. Images et sciences sociales, Multimédias en recherche*, no. 6, pp. 97–107, 1999.

[KAU 11] KAUFMANN J.-C., *L'entretien compréhensif*, Armand Colin, Paris, 2011.

[LAT 92] LATOUR B., *Aramis, ou l'amour des techniques*, La Découverte, Paris, 1992.

[MAL 03] MALONE R.E., "Distal nursing", *Social Science & Medicine*, vol. 56, pp. 2317–2326, 2003.

[MAR 10] MARTIN P., "Pouvoir pastoral, normalisation et soins infirmiers : une analyse foucaldienne", *APORIA*, vol. 2, no. 2, pp. 26–35, 2010.

[MAY 18] MAYERE A., "Patients projetés et patients en pratique dans un dispositif de suivi à distance : un 'travail des patients' recomposé", *Réseaux*, pp. 197–225, 2018.

[NOU 10] NOURY M., "Entre autonomie et responsabilité. L'individu au cœur des nouvelles stratégies de gouvernement de la santé", *Sociologie Santé*, no. 31, pp. 317–329, March, 2010.

[OUD 11] OUDSHOORN N., *Telecare Technologies and the Transformation of Healthcare*, Palgrave Macmillan, London, 2011.

[PIE 16] PIERRU F., "Le 'virage ambulatoire', de l'incantation à la pratique", *Soins*, vol. 61, no. 807, pp. 14–15, 2016.

[STR 97] STRAUSS A., FAGERHAUGH S., SUCZEK B. *et al.*, *Social Organization of Medical Work*, Transaction Publishers, New Brunswick, 1997.

PART 2

Care and Social Support: From Institutional Responses to Online Support

4

The Place of Care in the E-coordination of Home Care and Assistance

4.1. Introduction

According to the CGIET reports [PIC 12, PIC 13], the use of information and communication technologies (ICT) in health is becoming a major resource for cooperation between actors to enable empowerment, to compensate, maintain, prevent and facilitate links, and to energize the citizen. In spite of this, digital divides persist, particularly in the context of home care and care for people who are vulnerable or have lost autonomy. The need to incarnate, or even reincarnate, the care relationship through more "human", singular and interpersonal communication in the face of increased surveillance of health and illness, at a distance and mediatized by digital dispositives, is reopening the debate on the epistemological boundaries between a cure – understood as the act of caring – and care as a reflection of concern, attention and caring.

> CURE AND CARE. –
>
> Fleury [FLE 15] is particularly enlightening in highlighting the nuances between cure and care that define the act of treatment. A cure would therefore be an attempt to eradicate the disease, either through a treatment or an act of healing, regardless of the subject experiencing it. Care implies that the care is first considered in relation to the subject, the relationship with the doctor and the trust that is shown to him or her. Care and concern in the relationship are expressed in a feeling of equality in spite of dependence, even through an active vision of dependence in the sense of being able to "depend".

Chapter written by Géraldine GOULINET FITÉ.

Our proposal aims to examine the use of ICT in the home care context for elderly subjects weakened by chronic disease by studying their contribution(s) to the care process underlying the coordination of care and assistance pathways between professional home care workers.

To conduct our reflection, in section 4.2, we will present the issues related to the implementation of coordinated home care and assistance pathway.

This contextualization allows us to introduce section 4.3, which focuses on the communicational approach attributed to the concept of care. The use of the ethical and practical approach to care work is questioned (again) here with the deployment of remote health dispositives in service of the coordinated home care and home help pathway.

To illustrate our point, in section 4.4, we will present the case of the support network for the coordination of the *Escale Santé en Sud Gironde* (Nouvelle Aquitaine) process. We will detail the analysis of the digital uses carried out between the professional stakeholders and the support team via the PAACO-Globule digital coordination platform. The presentation of our results will be an opportunity to discuss the hypothesis that the socio-communicational added value of an e-coordination of home care and home help is based on its dual capacity to mediate and expose a collective care approach and practice.

4.2. Home care coordination issues

For several years now in France, the home care of elderly people made vulnerable by one or more diseases (chronic or degenerative) has led to a profound overhaul of the health, social and medico-social health model. The need for interprofessional cooperation is growing because of a twofold societal demand: that of more than 80% of French people wishing to age at home, and that of controlling and optimizing public health expenditure by promoting the shift to outpatient care [COT 02]. In order to go beyond these logics, since the 2000s French public policies have sought to integrate illness, disability and dependence into a common framework for action in solidarity and health programs, which have been constrained by the increasingly complex situations of elderly patients. This translates into the notion of a life course (life, health and care).

Chronologically, these initiatives are particularly highlighted by the Hospital, Patient, Health and Territory (*hôpital, patient, santé et territoire*, HPST) Act of July 21, 2009. This Act revolutionized the territorial organization of the healthcare system with the creation of the Regional Health Agencies (*agencies regionals de santé*, ARS), responsible for implementing regional healthcare policy by integrating a medico-social plan and a specific section for managing information systems. In this sense, it continues the paradigm shift brought about by the law of February 11, 2005 on the equal rights and opportunities, participation and citizenship of disabled people, which put an end to a purely medical approach to disability and, more broadly, to dependency [JAE 11].

Recently, the Adaptation to Aging Act of December 29, 2015, supplemented by the Healthcare System Modernization Act of January 26, 2016, illustrates the need to organize the coordinated care and assistance pathway for sick and elderly people, relying in particular on ICT. In this way, the logic of caring for dependency becomes consubstantial with that of preserving and maintaining well-being and autonomy. The need to ensure the care and assistance of elderly people at risk of loss of autonomy (*personnes âgées en risque de perte d'autonomie,* PAERPA) calls for a culture of aging well, based more on the Chronic Care Model [WAG 96] to prevent the risks associated with the onset of chronic disease.

From then on, cooperation in health care became a strategic tool for collective empowerment in the service of solidarity, which is no longer entrusted only to institutions, but also to home care and home help workers (citizens, family caregivers, professionals). In the field, professionals are experimenting with mediation [BON 97] to articulate their interventions, with a transfer of the operational public health center from the hospital to the patient's home [ROC 07]. With the development of coordination practices, interprofessional communication goes beyond simple interactions aimed solely at the circulation and transfer of information within a group to become an intermediate space, producing an improvement in the care of a person [DAV 03]. As a result, the third party (the person being cared for and/or their family and friends) becomes the subject of mediated communication (provided by means of communication) and the object of mediation between the various care providers and home help.

4.2.1. *Reconfigurations at home*

As a complex ecosystem, home care in France is legislated by two major ministerial bodies: on the one hand, the *Direction générale de l'offre de soins*, responsible for building and managing the provision of care, and, on the other hand, the *Direction générale de la cohésion sociale* (DGCS), responsible for designing, managing and evaluating public solidarity policies to promote social cohesion and support for people's autonomy. Through this national governance, the provision of home care and home help services is based on a composite structure made up of several types of operators (see Figure 4.1).

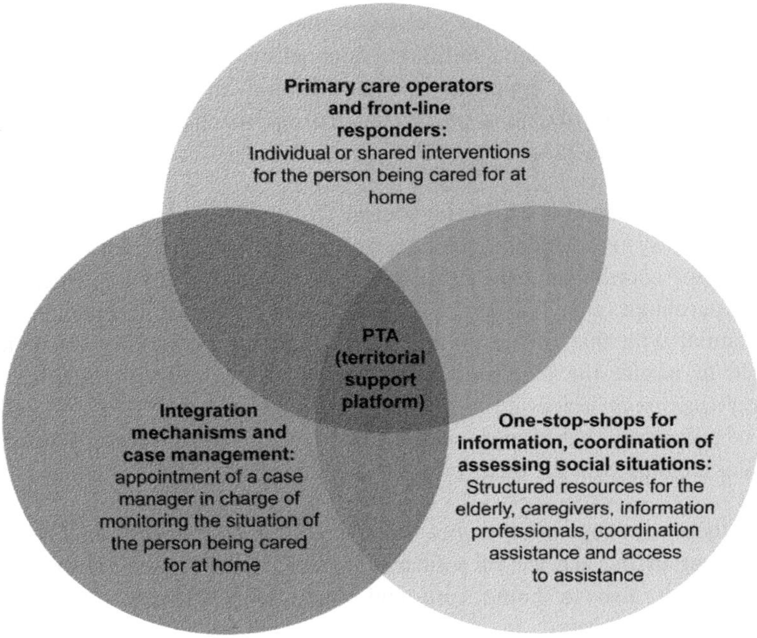

Figure 4.1. *Organizational ecosystem of home care and support services. For a color version of this figure, see www.iste.co.uk/cordelier/health.zip*

4.2.1.1. *Primary care and front-line help providers*

Primary care and front-line assistance providers include independent liberal professionals (doctors, nurses, pharmacists, physiotherapists, etc.) or those grouped together in an independent mutualized service: group practice, home nursing care service (*service de soins infirmiers à domicile*, SSIAD), home help and support service (*service d'aide et d'accompagnement à domicile*, SAAD), multi-purpose home help and care service (*service polyvalent d'aide et de soins à domicile*, SPASAD) or health center, health hub, etc.

In order to support the shift to outpatient care, the health sector has been developing incentives for interprofessional collaboration for several years by providing financial assistance for the creation of nursing homes or by promoting the implementation of cooperation protocols between professionals. In terms of social intervention, the referencing or even designation of home help services (*services d'aide à domicile*, SAAD) by the Departments aims to guarantee control of the quality of service offered by the providers and compliance with the terms and conditions of the allocation of social aid.

4.2.1.2. *Information and evaluation windows for social situations*

In order to improve access to information for the aging population, since 2001, each Department has had one or more local information points grouped together under the local information and coordination center (*centre local d'information et de coordination,* CLIC). Its role is to advise, inform and guide seniors and their families, as well as all professionals working with seniors, on the offers and services available in the area, and on the possible dispositives and assistance available.

In order to assess the need to allocate social assistance, the medico-social teams of the Departmental councils intervene at the request of the person or a coordinating operator. Their task is to determine the level of autonomy lost based on an evaluation grid[1], to draw up the assistance plan in consultation with the person and to inform him/her about the benefit and the remaining dependents.

4.2.1.3. *Integration and case management support dispositives for coordinated pathways*

Since 2014, the implementation of the coordinated pathway for the elderly has been based on the PAERPA dispositive (elderly people at risk of loss of autonomy – *personnes âgées en risque de perte d'autonomie*) and the MAIA method (action method for the integration of assistance and care services in the field of autonomy – *méthode d'action pour l'intégration des services d'aide et de soins dans le champ de l'autonomie*).

This organizational model is based on two axes: optimizing the coordination of the actors among themselves and providing an offer of integrated care and assistance services for people aged 60 and over, in complex situations requiring intensive long-term follow-up (including during hospitalization periods). This activity can be entrusted to a case manager, who is an expert and trained for the task, or to a coordination support team. They become the referent for complex situations with the attending physician, professionals working at home, the elderly person or his/her caregiver.

In order to harmonize and generalize the idea of a coordinated approach, the 2016 Healthcare System Modernization Act plans to link the health and medico-social services structurally in all territories through the implementation of a territorial

1 In France, the evaluation model used is based on the AGGIR grid (*Autonomie gérontologique et groupes iso-ressources* – gerontological autonomy and iso-resource groups). It measures the activities performed or not performed by the individual alone, and makes it possible to define "iso-resource groups", which bring together individuals with similar levels of need for assistance in performing essential acts in daily life.

support platform (*plateforme territoriale d'appui*, PTA). This platform will become the single coordination point for the individual care, assistance and health pathway of all users in vulnerable situations requiring regular and continuous monitoring between home and hospitalization episodes.

4.2.2. *From computerization to health informatization*

Traditionally, the use of information and communication technologies in health and social work has followed a dual logic. One, which is centuries old, consists of encoding and dematerializing material information supports (paper documents, care sheets, patient records, etc.). This is intrinsically linked to the history of the computerization of health and social work and is, first and foremost, part of a rational and managerial approach [ROM 08].

The other, more current since the advent of the Internet, conditions new configurations in the transmission and sharing of information. In the context of health care and home care, the arrival of the Internet is initiating a process of significant evolution, moving from computerization to *informationalization* [MIE 03, TIN 08], that is, an increase in info-communication flows within a network that has become reticular – between professionals, institutions and healthcare users in particular.

With him, professionals are invited to commit to a "collaborative approach enriched and facilitated by IT, greater completeness, security and reliability of information" around the sharing of administrative, social, medical and paramedical data on a situation [ROM 08].

> INFORMATIONALIZATION. –
>
> For the cited authors, informationalization is the result of the contemporary movement leading to the "information society", in which any data disseminated becomes a cognitive object of communication, increased by the development of computers and data processing, by globalization and by the arrival of the Internet. It differs from computerization, where the academic focus is on the study of computer tools perceived as communication machines.

If it formalizes and standardizes the information system (IS), its deployment quickly (re)sets the limits, and even the pitfalls of communication between institutions and categories of professionals, between the liberal and hospital sectors. The lack of standardization in the adoption of a common computer language for the various stakeholders does not make it possible to make systems interoperable. If, since 2004, under the impetus of public policies, *re-engineering* has been taking place to increase access to the social health network (*réseau social santé*, RSS) and the development of the shared medical record (*dossier médical partagé*, DMP), the integration of the social sector in this logic of informationalization also raises problems other than those of interfacing information systems with each other with a view to digital convergence.

It is the relationship *with* care and *of* care that is then (re)questioned through:

– the issue of trust in the circulation and security of data flows within the various information systems. This is why the French Digital Health Agency[2] (ASIP Santé) is in charge of building up and guaranteeing the digital trust space in France and abroad. Thanks to the implementation of directories and user identification and authentication dispositives, professionals can exchange health data with each other via secure health messaging (MSSanté);

– the challenge of extending the shared medical secrecy between health, medico-social and social professionals constituting a "care team". Indeed, the Health Act of January 2016 modifies certain provisions on professional secrecy by authorizing the sharing of information between professionals involved in patient care. The attending physician becomes the hub and has access to all the information contained in the DMP, including the history.

Consequently, the deployment of ICT in health care no longer serves only to digitize healthcare processes; made up of electronic networks for exchanging and sharing data, but they are rather becoming a means of supporting health as a common good for the benefit of all. By promoting the cooperation and inclusion of all, users, health professionals and social workers are no longer just subjects of this ecosystem but have become initiators in their own right.

This is all the more true in the context of aging at home, where the use of ICT juxtaposes the need for accompaniment, help and support to preserve well-being and maintain autonomy, thus ensuring a mediating function between the health and social fields.

The Rialle report [RIA 07] points out this particularity in its definition of *gerontechnologies*, which, according to it, call for a real paradigm shift. Service offers must go beyond the boundaries of the health and social field to be arranged according to needs in a systemic whole, integrating technologies as a *modus operandi* (diagnosis–treatment) in organizing the work of professionals and in the daily environment of the individual. A true functional revolution [FRAN 10], *gerontechnologies* are moving away from medical care and remote medicine

2 Created by the French Ministry of Solidarity and Health in 2009.

activities to promote remote health [LAS 09] organized around a coordinated e-path of care and assistance.

The legal framework for remote medicine is set out in the HPST law of July 21, 2009. It is defined as a form of remote medical practice using ICT, bringing one or more healthcare professionals, including necessarily a medical professional, into contact with each other or with a patient.

It enables a diagnosis to be made and a preventive or post-treatment follow-up for a patient at risk to be established, and makes it possible to request a specialized opinion, prepare a therapeutic decision, prescribe products, prescribe or perform services or procedures, or to monitor the condition of patients.

The application of remote medicine practices revolves around five medical acts:

– remote consultation, which allows a doctor to consult remotely with a patient, who in turn can be assisted in person by another health professional;

– remote expertise, which allows a physician to seek the opinion of one or more expert physicians based on elements of the patient's medical record;

– remote monitoring, which allows a doctor to remotely interpret the data necessary for medical follow-up in order to make decisions about his or her care;

– remote assistance, which allows a doctor to remotely assist another professional in the performance of a treatment;

– remote medical regulation as part of the response to the emergency call.

Box 4.1. *Focus on remote medicine*

The exchange and sharing of information between professionals in the home serves to optimize the coordination of the actors and to foster a collaborative culture to help, support and accompany the elderly and vulnerable persons.

GERONTECHNOLOGIES. –

This is an interdisciplinary academic and professional field that synthesizes gerontology and technology. It consists of creating technological environments in the service of health, housing, mobility, communication, leisure and work of the elderly with a view to developing innovative products and services aimed at satisfying, preventing, compensating, assisting and organizing the care of elderly people in situations of fragility, disability or dependency.

4.3. Impacts on the logic of care, roles and identities

4.3.1. *From cure to care*

Although efforts in articulation and coordination are obvious, these changes do not, *de facto*, lead to coherence in the modalities of intervention. In fact, the development of this culture of transversal care for all professionals remains determined by their institutional affiliations and the construction of certain professional values. The use of ICT has repercussions on individual and collective practices within health work organizations [BON 07], as well as those of social workers [MEY 15, MEY 17].

In this context, the lines of negotiation [BAS 86, STR 78] or even renegotiations at home are affected in terms of autonomy management, professional logic [DAM 99] shared in the values of care, between cure and care [BAU 13], and are subject to a certain injunction to participate in the digital world [PRO 17].

First in terms of autonomy, because this, in its idealized vision, is the bearer of an emancipatory and reflexive capacity on the part of the individual in the face of all forms of dependence. On its negative side, autonomy in health can be perceived as a normative injunction imposed on the individual, resulting in the mobilization of a certain "biographical activation" [BES 09], which, with regard to the elderly or the most deprived, raises the question of *capabilities*, that is, the opportunities, capacities of choice and resources offered to achieve this [SEN 10, pp. 239–253].

In terms of the values attributed to health care: the weakening of collective regulations and the rise of deinstitutionalization are changing the direction of action for this population. This produces, in terms of the approach to care, a distension of logics [MOL 09] in which autonomy becomes one of the main adjustment variables of "care giving" and "caretaking". In fact, considering that no one ever acts completely on their own, just as we are all vulnerable, the capacity to act according to the logic of self-care is based either on a vision of relational independence, centered on cooperation and reciprocity (logic of care), or on a managerial rationality of care, centered on the adequacy of supply to demand (logic of choice).

In order to distinguish the different ways of providing care, Saillant proposes approaching it according to the concepts of the cure (biomedical treatment, technical dimension of the therapeutic act) and of care, which becomes the expression of the support of a therapeutic action [SAI 99].

Also, behind this demarcation, the idea is to take care out of the private sphere and a moral disposition and to give it a political dimension, capable of making it a model of society [TRO 09] and a managerial aim for the organization [PES 12] around a "complex cultural construction and the tangible work of care" [TRO 09, p. 170].

In practice, the technical nature of the cure allows elderly people supported by a doctor at home to benefit from treatments and technical support adapted to their pathologies, while the practice of care ensures the framework of collective attention, concern and care. The whole formalizes a dynamic system specific to home care and assistance.

4.3.2. *Informational and communicational approach to care*

For information and communication sciences, every system has irreducible properties, which are attributed to the presence of relationships that unite the components.

As these evolve, relationships can change and the interactions between the system and its environment can vary. The information according to Laborit [DEG 76] allows this system to be structured. Communication formalizes the cognitive, psychological and social content [MEY 86], on the one hand, and becomes one of the modes of expression of the care relationship, on the other hand [FIS 99].

These postulates lead us to propose an info-communicational interpretation of care based on a model of the relational system that composes it.

The movement around personal medicine, which was championed by Tournier in 1940 [FRU 41] and then by Balint [BAL 60], emphasizes the affective and transferential dimension of the doctor–patient encounter. At the nursing level, both Watson's caring approach [WAT 99] and Fawcett's perceptual approach [FAW 96] emphasize that care is based on taking into account the person's point of view on his or her illness and experience in order to adjust the response to the situation in a concerted manner. Rogers [ROG 51], meanwhile, considers the physician to be a caregiver *par excellence*. Integrating the person-centered approach (PCA) into the professional practice of caregivers, he demonstrates the value of engaging in a helping relationship between the caregiver and the patient centered on congruence, active listening, non-judgment and empathy.

Regarding the liaison between the caregiver and the person receiving care, while long dissociated from health care, the prevalence of chronic disease and the aging of the population have greatly increased interest in the place and role of the caregiver (professional or natural) as a full-fledged provider. Over the past 20 years, a particularly fertile field of research has been developed with the work of Gagnon and Saillant [GAG 00, SAI 01] on the new responsibilities of home care and Joublin's work on proximology [JOU 05, JOU 10].

This conceptual evolution of the relationship follows the same trajectory as that of the philosophy of health and care in its ethical purpose (see Table 4.1).

	Medical ethics	**Care ethics**	**Ethics of care**
Ethical design	Conviction/responsibility	Commitment/attention	Human development
Key authors	Aristotle, Hippocrates	Ricoeur, Levinas, Canguilhem	Rawls, Sen, Nussbaum
Practical application	Clinical/public medicine	Caring–Nursing–Holding	Social, health, education, politics, etc.
Morality, deontology	Lack of wrongdoing	Good treatment	Wellness
Relationship with the body	Rationality Pragmatic Object of care	Subjectivity Sensitive Subject of care	Interdependence Sensitive Subject of care
Relationship to identity	Socialization	Subjectivation	Individuation
Info-communicational approach to the caregiver–patient encounter	Located disease Singular colloquium Interpersonal dyadic (doctor–patient)	Located health and illness Sharing experience Ecosystem of care (professional caregivers)	Located life-vulnerability Narration daily life Human ecosystem (beneficiaries-providers)

Table 4.1. *Conceptual specifications of the care relationship according to ethical approaches*

From the perspective of information and communication sciences, we conceive the relational system of care as a space for exchanges between providers (consisting of carers and helpers) and a beneficiary, with the duties intended to bring help, accompaniment and support to a vulnerable person. This is structured through the different communication logics [WAT 67] with the aim of improving well-being and a better understanding of the situation.

In order to grasp the meaning of the exchanges in this system, we have chosen to understand care as a systemic model of communication [MUC 04] shaped from three essential components: an affective dimension structured around attachment [BOW 08, WIN 65], a conative dimension based on the expression of trust [HOV 60, PHA 02] and a social dimension shaping identities and the places occupied in private and public spaces [SIN 98] (see Figure 4.2). The cognitive dimension is associated more with the information system structuring the circulation of exchanges. However, given the extension of the network of actors mandated to coordinate home care and home help, can this singular and interpersonal practice be carried out at the collective level, in an organized and mediatized manner through remote health dispositives?

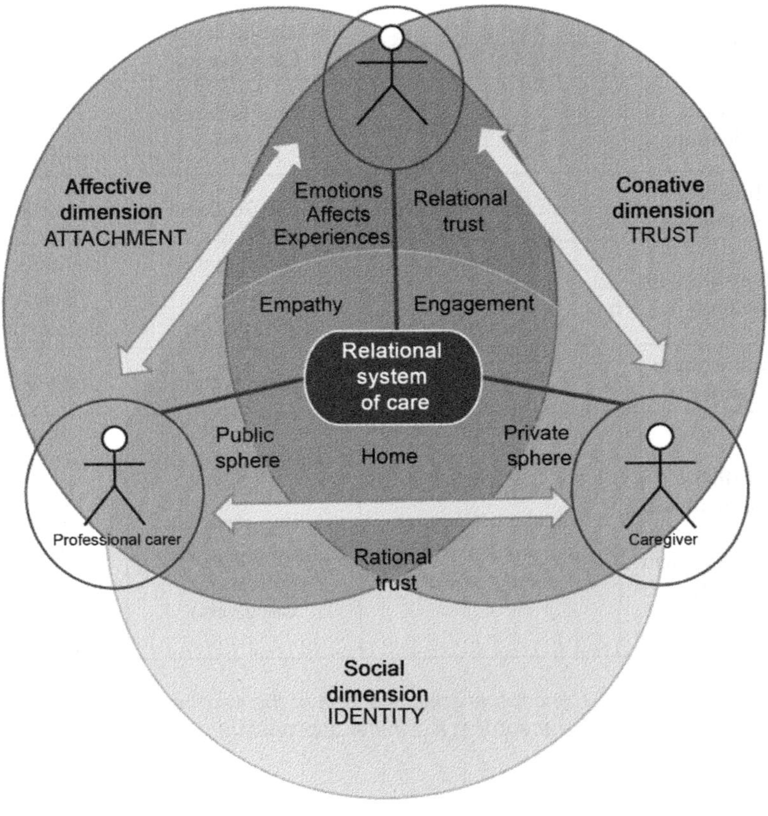

Figure 4.2. *Modeling the relational care system in home health care. For a color version of this figure, see www.iste.co.uk/cordelier/health.zip*

EXPOSURE. –

Based on the work of Davallon [DAV 03] and Jouet [JOU 00], we defined exposure as the means of producing social interactions through the use of a socio-technical dispositive. It differs from mediation, to which we attribute a capacity to create a practical instance of negotiation, a symbolic remedy between social actors, which, in our case study, aims to improve care.

The objective of section 4.4 is to develop this issue on the basis of a case study. The example chosen is the result of our investigations, carried out between July 2017 and June 2018 within the support network for the *Escale Santé* coordination in the South Gironde region and the use of the PAACO-Globule digital dispositive by the professionals in the support network and the home care and home help workers.

Through our observations, we will attempt to respond to the hypothesis that the added value of a digital coordination dispositive lies in its dual capacity to mediate the ethical and practical approach to care in favor of a common culture of interprofessional collaboration.

4.4. Uses and practices of the PAACO-Globule dispositive in a support network for the coordination of complex pathways in the South Gironde region

4.4.1. *Presentation of Escale Santé*

Escale Santé is a support structure for the coordination of complex and/or palliative care pathways. It is intended to develop a dynamic of networking between the city and the hospital, front-line health professionals and health, social and medico-social actors. Its aim is to promote home care for people weakened by illness and/or pathological aging. The team is composed of a director, a coordinating doctor, a medico-social secretary, three nurse coordinators, a social worker, a psychologist and an occupational therapist.

One of its missions is precisely to promote the use of ICT in facilitating the sharing and exchange of health/healthcare information in favor of remote health and remote medicine in proximity and focused on home care. Also, since 2012, *Escale Santé* has been using the PAACO-Globule dispositive as a "business" software and a communicating platform to exchange with professional caregivers and home help associated with the monitoring of complex situations.

Because of its mission statement, *Escale Santé* is one of the structures mandated to ensure the implementation of the South Gironde territorial support platform (*plateforme territoriale d'appui,* PTA). As an organizational dispositive, the PTA's vocation is to deploy collaborative digital solutions to promote the articulation of the work of actors in the field of home care and home help. The PAACO-Globule solution is designated at the regional level as the digital coordination tool required to ensure the operation of the PTAs (see Figure 4.3).

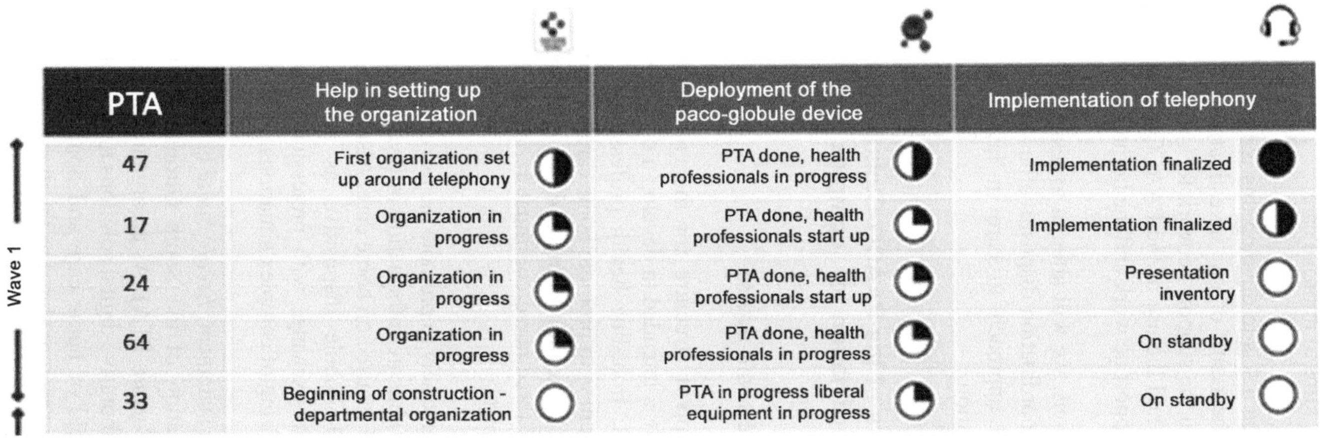

Figure 4.3. *Status of PAACO-Globule deployment by Departments (source: ARS Nouvelle Aquitaine, May 2018). For a color version of this figure, see www.iste.co.uk/cordelier/health.zip*

4.4.2. Presentation of the PAACO-Globule solution: functionalities and organizational framework

This secure and mobility-oriented communicative IT platform (computer, tablet and smartphone) is organized around three major functionalities:

– the management of a patient file that (re)traces personal and health data (life history, main diagnosis, reasons for the request, contact details of the staff and care network). Interoperability with most hospital information systems and business software promotes digital convergence with the pre-existing medical record (hospital and community medicine);

– a log of transmissions, notifications and SMS-type alerts in which images, sound and text files can be attached. The information-sharing of the note produced is systematically adjusted according to the level of confidentiality chosen by the sender (see Figure 4.4);

– collaborative tools, such as a task manager, shared calendars or an alert system.

The platform was launched in 2012, and initial feedback from field professionals (doctors, nurses connected) has been promising and positive. From 2013, the Regional Union of Private Doctors of Aquitaine *(Union régionale des médecins libéraux d'Aquitaine,* URPS ML) has supported the publisher (Ki-Labs) in the development of the solution, enhancing its added value in terms of ergonomics and functionalities:

> The web and smartphone versions of the system are able to centralize all the ingredients for efficient management of the shared patient file (administrative, educational, social, medical, personalized project, diary, liaison notebooks, letters, activity statistics) with communication tools (email, SMS, telephone, exchange of notes, photos, documents) in complete security. (*Journal de l'URPS*, no. 56, 2013, p. 10)

Taking advantage of the deployment of the shared medical record (DMP) and secure messaging (MSSanté) in Aquitaine, the *Groupement de coopération sanitaire* (GCS), Télésanté Aquitaine, which is responsible for supporting the widespread deployment of remote medicine and remote health solutions in the region, has been integrating this solution into its service package under the name PAACO-Globule (*Plateforme Aquitaine d'aide à la communication*) since 2014. This partnership enables the publisher to improve the conditions of interoperability between information systems (hospital and private sector) and increase its development potential. In addition, the testing in Bordeaux of the PAERPA dispositive (for elderly people at risk of loss of autonomy) and the successful application of the Santé-Landes project as part of the *Territoire de soins numériques* (TSN) program have been the formidable economic and organizational levers behind its widespread implementation since 2015 (see Figure 4.5).

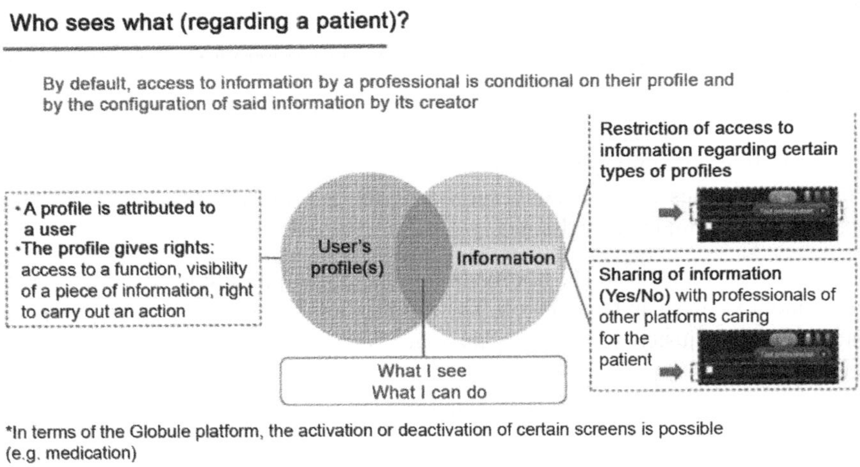

Figure 4.4. *Choice of the level of confidentiality with PAACO-Globule (source: ARS Nouvelle-Aquitaine, May 2018). For a color version of this figure, see www.iste.co.uk/cordelier/health.zip*

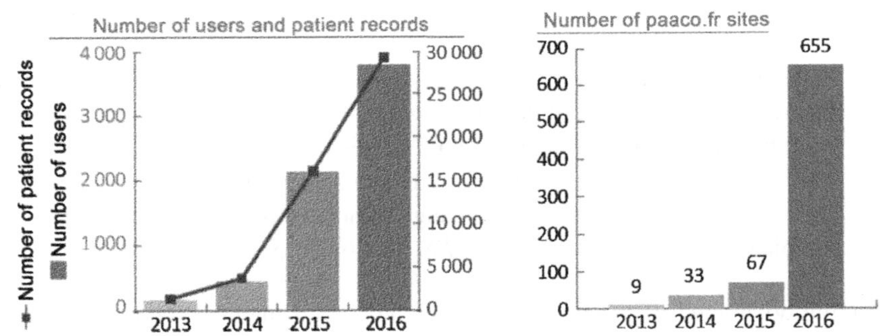

Figure 4.5. *Evolution of PAACO-Globule in Aquitaine (source: TSA activity report, 2016). For a color version of this figure, see www.iste.co.uk/cordelier/health.zip*

4.4.3. *Study design and presentation of results*

As researchers, we were involved in the team's work between July 2017 and June 2018. Our investigations were structured around two specific objectives: to characterize the reconfigurations of the coordination work in a context of digital mediatization, on the one hand, and to specify the numerical expressions of care in the coordination support activity of Escale Santé, on the other hand.

To do so, our qualitative research protocol was based on mixed methods combining:

– the distribution of a questionnaire to home care and home support workers in connection with *Escale Santé*. The survey was constructed from a non-representative convenience sample (N = 275);

– the conduct of semi-directive interviews conducted jointly by the *Escale Santé* support service team and respondents to the voluntary questionnaire (N = 20);

– the realization of ethnographic observations online of the notes from the PAACO-Globule transmission log from the *Escale Santé* platform (N = 50).

The data analysis for the semi-directive interviews and online ethnography were performed using NVivo software. The processing of the questionnaire survey was carried out using SPHINX.

In order to conduct our data processing plan in a comprehensive manner, the fields of analysis selected met two methodological and logical criteria: one was to meet the requirements of a construct validity specific to the case study [GAG 12] and the other was to be part of a process-based communication approach [MUC 04] (see Table 4.2).

The responses[3] from the sample (N = 275) have several significant characteristics.

While communication modes remain relatively traditional and bimodal (face-to-face/telephone) and reflect a cultural predominance of oral rather than written translation, the action of sharing and exchanging information on a patient's situation between professionals contributes, in representations, to producing coordination for 65.5% of respondents.

However, this perception is different from the reality of uneven regimes of cooperation between professions. Within the doctor–nurse pairing, this is in fact widespread (88.67% all the time, 49% often). On the other hand, engaging in personal cooperation and developing collaborative practices between medical, paramedical, social workers and home care professionals is much more irregular, if not non-existent, regardless of the means of communication used (see Figure 4.6).

3 A total of 53 responses were recorded, for a return rate of 19.2%.

	Questionnaire survey	Semi-directive interviews	Ethnographic observations online
Objective	Characterize the activity e-coordination	Report the care representation in e-coordination	Specify the exercise of care in e-coordination
Purpose	Identify communication functions of the sociotechnical environment of care		

Table 4.2. *Data processing plan*

This lack of consensus between the ideal and the reality of practices was particularly evident in the semi-directive interviews conducted with home care workers. They relate to practices instituted in an informal way, over time, and within a limited perimeter:

> Me, my podiatrist, the nurse and the psychologist who work in my home, when we talk to each other, we don't need anyone. A few satellite offices, nurses with whom we work a lot, it's the same thing. Coordination happens naturally, either by physically crossing each other and saying "by the way, madame machine…". (Excerpt from the doctor's interview)

> We don't go to the physiotherapist, we don't call the speech therapist, we don't call the podiatrist, if there is a problem we call the doctor, period, and we sort things out with the doctor. (Excerpt from the nurse's interview)

> When there are difficult cases, I go out into the field to find the nurse, that's it, to exchange and show and see a little bit of the reality of things. (Excerpt from the interview with the personal assistance service)

Even though cooperation and collaboration[4] [HEU 11] are seen as the main organizing functions of coordination for all respondents, they require (re)mediation, which a structure such as *Escale Santé* seems to embody in the eyes of the respondents.

---

4 According to the author, cooperation is defined as an *a priori* negotiated (rationalized) division of a task into actions that will be allocated (distributed) among individuals who will act relatively autonomously. Interactions are limited to organization, coordination and progress monitoring. The responsibility of each individual is limited to ensuring that the actions incumbent upon him/her are carried out: it is the progressive and coordinated succession of the fruit of each individual's action that makes it possible to achieve the objective.

Question 14 : Do you work with other professionals in monitoring patients at home?

	Often/All the time		Never/Rarely		Occasionally		Total	
	N	% cit.	N	% cit.	N	% cit.	N	% cit.
With the nurse	40	81.6%	1	2.0%	8	16.3%	49	100.0%
With the doctor	32	76.2%	4	9.5%	6	14.3%	42	100.0%
With home help professionals (carers, etc)	30	57.7%	4	7.7%	18	34.6%	52	100.0%
With the specialist doctor	20	38.5%	16	30.8%	16	30.8%	52	100.0%
With the pharmacist	18	34.6%	14	26.9%	20	38.5%	52	100.0%
With rehabilitation specialists and equipment (physiotherapists, occupational therapists, etc)	18	34.6%	15	28.8%	19	36.5%	52	100.0%
With social services professionals	18	34.6%	20	38.5%	14	26.9%	52	100.0%
With carers	11	21.6%	21	41.2%	19	37.3%	51	100.0%
With mental health nurses	8	15.7%	27	52.9%	16	31.4%	51	100.0%
Total	195	43.0%	122	26.9%	136	30.0%	453	

Some conditions have been grouped

Figure 4.6. *Status of interprofessional cooperation relationships. For a color version of this figure, see www.iste.co.uk/cordelier/health.zip*

What gives rise to a desire to cooperate and collaborate is the need for help, support and accompaniment when the doctor/nurse pairing, whose practice is mainly focused on the technical aspect of care or cure, reaches the limits of their ability to manage a complex situation at home.

In the questionnaire survey, this translates in two specific ways: first, through the mandate given to *Escale Santé* and, second, in the qualification of the professional values it conveys to the respondents. Indeed, because of its support function for coordination, *Escale Santé* is unanimously perceived as a productive entity of collective "caretaking" (50.94% strongly agree and 49.05% agree).

Indeed, two axes emerge from the survey: one, info-communication, the other in relation to moral dispositions of attention and solicitude. In the first, informational practices are useful means of accessing information in order to better work together in a given context. In this respect, they serve relational functions associated with the *Escale Santé* mode of organization (among the groups of words proposed, the item "cooperation, communication, relationship" is cited by 39%). The second pole shows the extent to which moral dispositions underlie the acts of communication and involvement in informational practices (the two items "trust, tolerance, consultation" and "listening, empathy, concern" are respectively cited by 17%, i.e. a total representativeness of 73% for these three items).

In short, these two vectors confer on *Escale Santé* a statutory recognition in which the Network appears as an effective agent of care, mainly at the service of the actors of the cure. The aim is to optimize the work of prescribing care and assistance and to improve the vigilance and individual and collective monitoring of the professionals associated with the health and personal care pathway.

In the digital traces of *Escale Santé*'s activities recorded from our online ethnographic observation, this is reflected in its performative work of written translations of the activity carried out. Also called "working aloud" [BON 13], this info-communication practice is mediatized in the PAACO-Globule logbook as "communication notes" in the form of secure notes (chat) that the members of the *Escale Santé* team then share with the professional teams in charge of providing care and assistance (in the sense of a cure) to the beneficiary.

However, this digital writing work shows the existence of an extremely codified lexical grammar used to categorize the content and purposes of the logbook notes transmitted to professionals associated with care, according to the function and role of the writer. The digital productions of the coordinating physician and the director of Escale Santé, when they are shared, are therefore systematically notified in red.

09/10/17 (16 months) – XXX Christine (nurse), coordinator
Confidentiality, Cell group

Call made to the nurse's office:
Objective of the call: give an update on the development of the situation and inform them of the assessment visit date.
Left them a message inviting them to call me back

Call made to retirement home XXX:
Agreement made to schedule an assessment visit on Friday 13 October at 10am, visit made by Christine + Clémence + IDE structure

Call made to M. XXX, son:
I confirmed the assessment date visit. He sent to us via email a table outlining a schedule for different professionals who could help Mrs X should she return home.

Figure 4.7. *Example of notes from the logbook. For a color version of this figure, see www.iste.co.uk/cordelier/health.zip*

This color-coded differentiation allows the expected content to be immediately associated with it: that of reporting on decisions taken on a situation, either as a result of internal meetings within the Escale Santé team or during consultation meetings conducted with associated professionals (see Figure 4.8).

15/01/18 (13 months) XXX Clémence (director/coordinator), **Socio-educational framework.**
Confidentiality, Doctors + carers

Staff from 15/01/18
Christelle D assessed Mrs X's situation on 12/01 at the rental she is staying at. Current conditions are poor (no insulation and little heating. Mrs X is sleeping on a camp bed).
Her medical situation is relatively stable for the moment but she has social problems +++.
Mrs X is still independent. She is having a course of chemotherapy at the sud Gironde de Langon hospital.
She has found a new doctor to treat her locally: Dr B.
Mrs X was hospitalized at the Bazas follow-up and rehabilitative care center where a request for her protection was made. Mrs X refused.
History of a complex life which was discussed. Necessity for orientation towards a social assistant from MDSI/housing problem.

– CAT:
– Christelle carried out the PPS
– Document passed to the "palliative situation" unit
– Laure C. made contact with the hospital's social assistant to establish communication and create a link with the MDSI social service

Figure 4.8. *Example of notes from Escale Santé staff. For a color version of this figure, see www.iste.co.uk/cordelier/health.zip*

In its lexical form, this type of note follows more of a cure logic in which the elements of medical diagnosis (history, pathologies, treatments, state of care), the reasons for inclusion (social, psychological, nursing, functional rehabilitation) and decision-making are mainly found.

In fact, their sharing is almost always limited to the doctor/nurse pairing responsible for providing more technical care. Basically, they serve two purposes: one internal to the network as a sociotechnical dispositive organizing the management and distribution of tasks within the team, and the other external as a communication process organizing coordination in its negotiation dynamics (decisions are shared).

Insofar as their function is not to engage in dialog but to “report” on the coordination work, the “discussion thread” constituted through the digital notes produced by the entire *Escale Santé* multidisciplinary team calls for very few comments in PAACO-Globule by the associated care and assistance professionals.

However, it is through the modes of writing and distribution chosen by the team that these notes are similar to a work of care in the eyes of the professionals interviewed. The lexical structure of their notes prescribes several info-communication modalities aiming at recognition (of oneself, of the other), in the sense of Honneth [HON 04], making it possible to make the relational work of care visible.

This is reflected in the logbook by:

1) a transcript of all communication acts (incoming and outgoing calls, document transmissions, email extracts, physical meeting, etc.) aimed at qualifying the contacts and characterizing the content of interpersonal exchanges on the situation;

2) a systematic dating of all actions and an effort to (re)contextualize the chronology of the shared notes in order to account for intercurrent events and the coordination follow-up carried out;

3) an asserted choice for narrative expression (style of writing and explanation of written numerical notes) that makes it possible to translate the intersubjectivity of the relational work carried out with the beneficiary (valorization of the interactions with him/her and his/her entourage, expression of his/her feelings, emotions, etc.). In addition, each note written by the team endeavors to reflect the identity and corporeality of the person (systematic use of *Mr* or *Ms* in all the notes, recurrent reminders of elements of his or her life history and/or social, economic, psychological or cognitive environment making it possible to individualize the remarks), the same elements that risk being “erased” by the use of digital technology [LEB 14].

Organized on a daily basis, this electronic transcription work contributes to the digital use of the dispositive which, in terms of the technical and social acceptability of the *Escale Santé* team and of the care and assistance professionals who commission it, is built around two functions: a receptive function with an informational vocation (in reading) and an expressive function with a communicational aim (in writing).

This is also true of the responses from the corpus of connected professionals (representing 39.62% of respondents) who mainly develop a digital receptive function that is more than expressive. As a result, their uses are concentrated on an activity of consulting the logbook in order to stay informed of the intercurrent events of a situation (71.42% cite “all the time” and “often”).

For these users, the dispositive goes beyond the simple normative function of information transmissions to become a living documentary and documented space for monitoring the pathway capable of providing a global, systemic and singular vision of each situation:

> Once my work day is over, I can think about my patients and then take stock by looking at the bubbles, sometimes I even go back to the very beginning to remind myself a little bit of the evolution of things, which I find very interesting. (Excerpt from the doctor’s interview)

> It’s for clarifying, especially for following the development, it’s really where we talk about the patient as a whole because sometimes under lumbar complaints, for example, it’s family histories and sometimes stories of rape, etc., and that I can’t manage all alone! (Excerpt from the doctor’s interview)

When they are in an expressive contribution process of using logbook notes, this is first to share the miniature patient record (61.90% cite “all the time” and “often”) and then the letters, reports and forms (57.14% cite “all the time” and “often”).

For *Escale Santé*, the perceived usefulness of these textual discussions is its capacity to make visible the intangible capital of information and communication that serves coordination.

4.5. Conclusion

We see that despite the incentive programs to optimize the coordination of care and home care pathways, our work leads us to observe that this work of coordinating professionals around a patient is not a natural phenomenon. It is a construction, a complex process resulting from interprofessional collaborative practices that our various investigations have sought to determine through the functional analysis they produce (utility, use, constraints, esteem).

In the context of digital exposure, this case study shows that the use of PAACO-Globule, as a business software, becomes the instrument through which *Escale Santé* legitimizes its mission of coordination support according to three logics:

– a logic of management of information flows (processing and distribution of information);

– a relational logic (animation of the beneficiary's socio-professional network);

– a logic of mediation (as an intermediary mandated to conciliate all the parties involved in a complex situation).

The info-communication activity produced by *Escale Santé* serves as a traceability system that enhances the ethics and practice of care with respect to home care and home help workers.

In this respect, and from our disciplinary perspective, the results of our work corroborate the thesis of the situated acceptance approach [BOB 16], which consists of evaluating the appropriation of uses based on a triangulation of the different dimensions that make it up (relational, organizational, identity, professional). From our point of view, the study of info-communication practices offers the opportunity to identify their contours.

Through them, the collective exercise of care appears to be a certain approach factor that makes it possible to make the technology acceptable because it is

> benevolent and empowering for the individual and for their activity, insofar as it allows them to develop their practices and skills […] and that finally it contributes to putting their (publicized) work into debate, becoming an object of conflictuality, both reflexive and constructive for them and for others. [BOB 16]

The term "literacy" refers to the knowledge and skills in reading, writing, speaking (or other means of communication) and numeracy that enable people to function and participate in society. Adapted to health – health literacy – like other forms of literacy (e.g. digital literacy), it reflects the contextual nature of its field.

Its most recent definition emphasizes its system of representation composed of the knowledge, motivation and skills needed to "access, understand, evaluate and apply health information; to make judgments and decisions about health care, prevention and health promotion, with the goal of maintaining and promoting quality of life throughout life" [SØR 12].

There is general agreement across international studies that low literacy levels are associated with a lower participation in prevention activities, a higher prevalence of health risk factors, less effective communication with healthcare professionals, a limited understanding of prescriptions and increased adverse drug reactions, limited autonomy in chronic disease management, increased hospitalization and readmission, and increased healthcare costs [BER 11, EAS 10]. As a result, it is now seen as a lever for improving the quality of care and combating health inequalities. The best known tool for measuring it is the Health Literacy Questionnaire (HLQ).

Patients' digital literacy takes into consideration the skills to identify useful and necessary information, to locate, evaluate and use it in a problem-solving process. This set can be presented as a series of skills that allows the patient to find his or her way around the digital health ecosystem.

Three levels of complementary skills [VEN 06] are identified to build the foundation of a digital culture:

– instrumental skills related to the handling of hardware and software. They primarily cover the operational skills that are part of basic know-how;

– structural or informational skills that relate to the new way of entering online content, that is, searching, selecting, understanding, evaluating, processing information;

– strategic skills. They concern the ability to use information proactively, give it meaning in its own living environment and make decisions to act on its environment. They support goal-oriented behavior.

This leads us to establish a framework for the digital capabilities of users, which, with reference to the idea of patient empowerment, establishes literacy as a lever for individual and collective action to empower people to act and express democracy in health [DUM 17]. In this sense, the accessibility of e-health for patients would be a means of rebalancing the caretaker–patient relationship by giving patients access to information and knowledge hitherto held by health professionals. From a more critical point of view, this capacity raises new spheres of responsibility for the individual in his or her relationship to health promotion based on injunctions rather than freedom of choice [COL 13].

Box 4.2. *Literacy, digital literacy of patients, digital empowerment of users*

4.6. References

[BAL 60] BALINT M., VALABREGO J.-P., *Le médecin, son malade et la maladie*, Payot, Paris, 1960.

[BAS 86] BASZANGER I., "Les maladies chroniques et leur ordre négocié", *Revue française de sociologie*, pp. 3–27, 1986.

[BER 11] BERKMAN N., SHERIDAN S., DONAHUE K.E. *et al.*, "Low health literacy and health outcomes: An updated systematic review", *Annals of Internal Medicine*, vol. 155, no. 2, pp. 97–107, 2011.

[BES 09] BESSIN M., "Parcours de vie et temporalités biographiques : quelques éléments de problématique", *Informations Sociales*, no. 6, pp. 12–21, 2009.

[BOB 16] BOBILLIER CHAUMON M.-E., "L'acceptation située des technologies dans et par l'activité : premiers étayages pour une clinique de l'usage", *Psychologie du travail et des organisations*, vol. 22, no. 1, pp. 4–21, 2016.

[BON 97] BONAFE-SCHMITT J., "Les médiations", *Communication et organisation*, no. 11, 1997.

[BON 07] BONNEVILLE L., GROSJEAN S., "Les défis que soulève l'informatisation de la pratique médicale sur le plan de l'innovation technologique", *Canadian Journal of Communication*, vol. 32, no. 3, 2007.

[BOW 08] BOWLBY E., *Attachment: Volume One of the Attachment and Loss Trilogy*, Random House, New York, 2008.

[COT 02] COTE D., *Le virage ambulatoire : défis et enjeux*, Presses de l'Université du Québec, Quebec, 2002.

[COL 13] COLLETTE K., ROUSSEAU J., "Littératie et responsabilité en santé", *Globe*, no. 16, pp. 107–131, 2013.

[DAM 99] D'AMOUR D., SICOTTE C., LEVY R., "L'action collective au sein d'équipes interprofessionnelles dans les services de santé", *Sciences sociales et santé*, vol. 17, no. 3, pp. 67–94, 1999.

[DAV 03] DAVALLON J., "La médiation : la communication en procès", *Médias et information*, no. 19, pp. 37–59, 2003.

[DEG 76] DE GUISE J., "Henri Laborit, la nouvelle grille pour décoder le message humain, 1974", *Communication. Information médias théories*, vol. 1, no. 1, pp. 393–400, 1976.

[DES 98] DE SINGLY F., "Individualisme et lien social", *Lien social et politiques*, no. 39, pp. 33–45, 1998.

[DUM 17] DUMEZ H., MINVIELLE H., "L'e-santé rend-elle la démocratie sanitaire pleinement performative ?" *Systèmes d'information & management*, vol. 22, no. 1, pp. 9–37, 2017.

[EAS 10] EASTON P., ENTWISTLE V., WILLIAMS B., "Health in the 'hidden population' of people with low literacy, a systematic review of the literature", *BMC Public Health*, vol. 10, no. 1, p. 459, 2010.

[FAW 96] FAWCETT J., "On the requirements for a metaparadigm: An invitation to dialogue: Commentary", *Nursing Science Quarterly*, vol. 9, no. 3, pp. 94–97, 1996.

[FIS 99] FISCHER G.-N., "Le concept de relation en psychologie sociale", *Recherche en soins infirmiers*, vol. 56, pp. 4–11, 1999.

[FLE 15] FLEURY C., "Le care-cure, chronique philo du 20 mars 2015", *L'Humanité*, available at: https://www.humanite.fr/le-care-cure-568910, 2015.

[FRA 10] FRANCO A., RIALLE V., "Perte d'autonomie et maintien à domicile", *Esprit*, no. 7, pp. 85–92, 2010.

[FRU 41] FRUTIGER P., *Médecine de la personne*, Delachaux et Niestlé, Neuchâtel and Paris, 1941.

[GAG 00] GAGNON É., SAILLANT F., *De la dépendance et de l'accompagnement : soins à domicile et liens sociaux*, Presses de l'Université Laval, Quebec, 2000.

[HON 04] HONNETH A., "Visibilité et invisibilité, sur l'épistémologie de la reconnaissance", *Revue du MAUSS*, no. 1, pp. 137–151, 2004.

[JAE 11] JAEGER M., *Usagers ou citoyens ? De l'usage des catégories en action sociale et médico-sociale*, Dunod, Paris, 2011.

[JOU 00] JOUËT J., "Retour critique sur la sociologie des usages", *Réseaux*, no. 100, pp. 389–521, 2000.

[JOU 05] JOUBLIN H., *Réinventer la solidarité de proximité : manifeste de proximologie*, Albin Michel, Paris, 2005.

[JOU 10] JOUBLIN H., *Le proche de la personne malade et l'univers des soins*, Érès, Toulouse, 2010.

[LAS 09] LASBORDES P., La télésanté : un nouvel atout au service de notre bien-être, Un plan quinquennal éco-responsable pour le déploiement de la télésanté en France, available at: http://www.ladocumentationfrancaise.fr/var/storage/rapports-publics/094000539.pdf, 2009.

[LEB 14] LE BRETON D., "Le corps entre significations et informations", *Hermès, La Revue*, no. 1, pp. 21–30, 2014.

[MEY 86] MEYRIAT J., "Information vs communication ?", in LAULAN A.-M. (ed.), *L'espace social de la communication. Concepts et théories*, Retz, CNRS, Paris, 1986.

[MEY 15] MEYER C., "La santé, le social : débats anciens et enjeux actuels", *Revue de la recherche en travail social*, no. 143, p. 59, 2015.

[MEY 17] MEYER V., *Transition digitale, handicaps et travail social*, LEH Édition, Bordeaux, 2017.

[MIE 03] MIEGE B., "La contribution des industries de la culture, de l'information et de la communication à l'informationnalisation et à la globalisation", *Questions de communication*, no. 3, pp. 211–229, 2003.

[MOL 09] MOL A., *Ce que soigner veut dire*, Presses des Mines, Paris, 2009.

[MUC 04] MUCCHIELLI A., *Étude des communications : approche systémique dans les organisations*, Armand Colin, Paris, 2004.

[PES 12] PESQUEUX Y., "De l'engagement au care", *Question(s) de management*, no. 2, pp. 107–118, 2012.

[PHA 02] PHANUEL D., "Confiance dans les soins et soin de la confiance : la réponse relationnelle", *Politiques et management public*, vol. 20, no. 4, pp. 115–132, 2002.

[PIC 12] PICARD R., DESHAYES C., Rapport "Bien Vivre grâce au numérique", Ministère de l'Économie et des Finances, Conseil général de l'Économie, de l'Industrie, de l'Énergie et des Technologies (C.G.E.I.E.T.), Paris, available at: www.ethique-cancer.fr/files/file_fields/2015/11/16/rapportbienvivregraceaunumerique.pdf, 2012.

[PIC 13] PICARD R., DESHAYES C., STUCHLIK J.-F., Rapport : prospective organisationnelle pour un usage performant des technologies nouvelles en Santé, Ministère de l'Économie et des Finances, Conseil général de l'Économie, de l'Industrie, de l'Énergie et des Technologies (C.G.E.I.E.T.), Paris, available at: https://www.economie.gouv.fr/files/files/directions_services/cge/prospective-technologies-sante.pdf, 2013.

[PRO 17] PROULX S., "L'injonction à participer au monde numérique", *Communiquer. Revue de communication sociale et publique*, no. 20, pp. 15–27, 2017.

[RIA 07] RIALLE V., Technologies nouvelles susceptibles d'améliorer les pratiques gérontologiques et la vie quotidienne des malades âgés et de leur famille, Report, Ministère de la Santé et des Solidarités, Paris, 2007.

[ROC 07] ROCHE F., "Le rapport du CSTS sur l'articulation du sanitaire et du social", *Vie sociale*, no. 1, pp. 87–95, 2007.

[ROG 51] ROGERS C., "A theory of personality and behavior", *Client-Centered Therapy: Its Current Practice, Implications, and Theory*, Houghton Mifflin, Boston, 1951.

[ROM 08] ROMEYER H., "TIC et santé : entre information médicale et information de santé", *Tic&société*, vol. 2, no. 1, 2008.

[ROS 60] ROSENBERG M.J., HOVLAND Y., HOVLAND C. *et al.*, "Cognitive, affective and behavioral components of attitudes", in ROSENBERG M.J. (ed.), *Attitude Organisation and Change: An Analysis of Consistency Among Attitude Components*, Yale University Press, New Haven, 1960.

[SAI 99] SAILLANT F., "Femmes, soins domestiques et espace thérapeutique", *Anthropologie et sociétés*, vol. 23, no. 2, pp. 15–39, 1999.

[SAI 01] SAILLANT F., GAGNON É., "Responsabilité pour autrui et dépendance dans la modernité avancée, le cas de l'aide aux proches", *Lien social et politiques*, no. 46, pp. 55–69, 2001.

[SEN 10] SEN A., *The Place of Capability in a Theory of Justice. Measuring Justice: Primary Goods and Capabilities*, Cambridge University Press, Cambridge, 2010.

[SØR 12] SØRENSEN K.,VAN DEN BROUCKE S., FULLAM J. *et al.*, "Health literacy and public health: A systematic review and integration of definitions and models", *BMC Public Health*, vol. 12, no. 1, p. 80, 2012.

[STR 78] STRAUSS A.L., *Negotiations: Varieties, Contexts, Processes, and Social Order*, Jossey-Bass, 1978.

[TIN 08] TINE M.-A., "Une critique du processus d'informationnalisation du système de santé français", *Tic&société*, vol. 2, no. 1, 2008.

[TRO 09] TRONTO J., MAURY H., *Un monde vulnérable, pour une politique du "care"*, La Découverte, Paris, 2009.

[VAL 06] VALENDUC G., VENDRAMIN P., "Fractures numériques, inégalités sociales et processus d'appropriation des innovations", *Terminal*, pp. 137–154, 2006.

[WAG 96] WAGNER E.H., AUSTIN B.T., VON KORFF M., "Organizing care for patients with chronic illness", *The Milbank Quarterly*, pp. 511–544, 1996.

[WAT 67] WATZLAWICK P., BEVELAS J., JACKSON D., *Pragmatics of Human Communication*, W.W. Norton & Company, New York, 1967.

[WAT 99] WATSON J., *Nursing: Human Science and Human Care: A Theory of Nursing*, Jones & Bartlett Learning, Burlington, 1999.

[WIN 65] WINNICOTT D., *The Maturational Processes and the Facilitating Environment: Studies in the Theory of Emotional Development*, The Hogarth Press and the Institute of Psycho-analysis, London, 1965.

5

Breast Cancer Prevention Online in a Crisis of Confidence Context: From Medical–Technical Discourse to Social Support

5.1. Introduction

Prevention policies and actions in France are facing several upheavals owing to a more global health crisis. Defining a health crisis means analyzing an unusual emerging event that goes beyond the scope of routine alert management, in terms of its scope, severity or media coverage, and may require coordination with many highly involved players. We can thus talk about and analyze phenomena related to the crisis of informational and communicational legitimacy or the questioning of expertise. A climate of mistrust towards health experts and institutions has gradually been established in France, following various political and health affairs, and conflicts of interest, as well as fears raised by the emergence of diseases, pathologies or viruses that are out of control. We are also witnessing certain pharmaceutical company scandals (Médiator, Vioxx, etc.) and the proliferation of consumer products considered carcinogenic. At the same time, forms of individualizing health practices and life choices are developing, such as the refusal of vaccinations [OLL 17] or the call for alternative medicine [ROM 13]. Some practitioners [SAO 09] speak of a crisis of confidence among citizens with respect to the healthcare system. This crisis of confidence is not without consequences for the online info-communication practices of patients and healthcare professionals.

Chapter written by Dorsaf OMRANE and Pierre MIGNOT.

Since 2016, our research has focused on the info-communication practices of the organizations, health practitioners and population concerned with breast cancer prevention. We will try to answer the following question: in a context of crisis of confidence linked to the health environment in general and to the polemics around breast cancer screening in particular, what are the perceptions of the population concerned with regard to institutional and medico-technical discourse? Indeed, our approach is focused on what the population concerned by breast cancer thinks about prevention campaigns and their online info-communication practices. In addition to the practices related to compliance or controversy [OMR 18], those related to online social relationships are omnipresent and cross-cutting, and question us on the challenges of online prevention systems.

INFO-COMMUNICATION PRACTICES. –

By "practices", we mean "the habits of doing", in the sense of Jacques Perriault [PER 89], which combine both the knowledge and representations that make it possible to understand and apply them according to the relevant situation. The practices therefore "cover not only the use of techniques but also the behaviors, attitudes and representations of individuals that relate to the tool" [JOU 93]. Indeed, these info-communication practices are diverse and the sources are varied. Audiences are informed by the combined action of associations and traditional media, which now treat health topics from a critical angle [ROM 13], as well as, more recently, by the exponential development of online health information and the use of digital devices [THO 12a].

The observation and content analysis of our field revealed two mechanisms of trust between the population affected by cancer and the actors in prevention campaigns (here, doctors, associations and institutions): an "impersonal" mechanism based on the skills and standardization conveyed in the prevention campaigns and an "interpersonal" mechanism based on social support between the population affected by breast cancer, through which we find their life stories and experiential knowledge.

In section 5.2, we will first propose understanding the context of the crisis of confidence linked to the historical, organizational and communicational specificities of breast cancer prevention through its mechanisms and actors. Then, we will present our research methodology (section 5.3) and the main results of our online ethnographic study on the info-communication practices of the population concerned with regard to prevention discourses (section 5.4). Here, we will only discuss practices that fall under the heading of online social support.

Defining compliance is not an easy task, as there is no consensus on it. Initially, it was used as a synonym for conformity. However, this notion of conformity is part of a more legal vocabulary, whereas the notion of compliance is foreign to French legal culture: "Modern French legal culture was built on the idea of legality, i.e. on the idea that there are rules that order conduct, dictate prohibitions and threaten those who violate them with a sentence, pronounced at the end of a trial." [GAU 19] Compliance is less vertical than this notion of conformity. It induces a much stronger notion of adaptation on the part of individuals. It requires acceptance by all actors. Here, we are faced with a form of collective acceptance that is also structured around a rule, a standard. Compliance here means accepting the screening method and treatment proposed, trusting the doctor's knowledge and normality (age, family precedents, etc.).

If we are interested in this dispute, we can take the two approaches of the *Centre national de ressources textuelles et lexicales* (French National Center of Textual and Lexical Resources)[1]:

– the first is "a discussion between persons on a point of contention, a quarrel resulting from rival claims". It is indeed a public debate on a societal issue;

– the second is about "questioning preconceived ideas, institutions, the social order, systematically criticizing the established order". The latter also makes it possible to think of a space for the norm and of questioning these norms.

The question of controversy is, therefore, at the same time a space for debate and also for questioning public health policies. As Caroline Ollivier-Yanniv evokes it: "Public health has not ceased to be publicly called into question, through controversies that question the relationship between public action, political responsibility, biomedical expertise, economic interests and the pharmaceutical sector's capacity to influence – colloquially and pejoratively referred to as Big Pharma" [OLL 15]. Breast cancer screening is no exception to this challenge.

Box 5.1. *Compliance and controversy*

5.2. Prevention and crisis context

Before moving on to the presentation of the context, it is appropriate to clarify beforehand the meaning we attribute to "prevention".

PREVENTION.–

Prevention is the set of measures aimed at avoiding or reducing the number and severity of illnesses or accidents; moreover, contrary to what is commonly known, prevention concerns the period during and after illness. For this study, we have

1 https://www.cnrtl.fr/definition/controverse.

chosen to refer to the distinction proposed by the World Health Organization (WHO) of primary, secondary and tertiary prevention. Primary prevention includes all acts intended to reduce the incidence of a disease in a population, and thus to reduce the risk of new cases appearing. It involves individual prevention measures (personal hygiene, nutrition, physical and sports activities, vaccinations, etc.) and collective prevention measures (distribution of drinking water, waste disposal, safe food, vaccinations, home and workplace hygiene). This traditional conception of prevention inevitably leads to a very broad program to improve the quality of life and reform social institutions. Secondary prevention aims to reduce the prevalence and the time of development of a disease in a population. It takes into account the early detection and treatment of the first infections. Tertiary prevention includes all acts intended to reduce the prevalence of chronic disabilities or recurrences in a population, thus minimizing functional disabilities resulting from the disease. This concept extends prevention to the field of rehabilitation and seeks to promote professional and social reintegration.

During our study, we first tried to identify and analyze the different dimensions of prevention on the association's Facebook page "Breast cancer, let's talk about it!" ("*Le cancer du sein, parlons-en!*" in the original French), and then to analyze the different contents and interactions. Even if our study was initially interested in primary and then secondary prevention related to breast cancer screening, we realized that content related to social ties is omnipresent in the exchanges around any type of prevention. This is why we chose not to limit ourselves solely to primary and secondary prevention for this work.

Breast cancer prevention is facing a crisis, which is reflected in the fact that organized screening rates have stagnated at 52% since 2008[2], that is, four years after the launch of the organized screening program, which is the main prevention technique in France. More and more people are speaking out against screening techniques and are calling for prevention that takes into account socio-environmental factors in the fight against cancer [MEN 10]. Paradoxically, we note a multiplicity of actors involved in breast cancer prevention campaigns, whether institutional, private or associative.

5.2.1. *The breast cancer prevention in question: its system and players*

Despite its protean nature, the basis of breast cancer prevention today is based on a collective injunction for early detection developed within the framework of

2 http://www.e-cancer.fr/Professionnels-de-sante/Depistage-et-detection-precoce/Depistage-du-cancer-du-sein/Le-programme-de-depistage-organise#toc-le-d-pistage-organis-en-quelques-chiffres.

organized screening. Communication and promotional campaigns and actions for this system are increasingly being carried out by a variety of players. In spite of their progressive evolution since the beginning of the 20th century, the systems and the players involved still raise many questions today.

5.2.1.1. *Breast cancer prevention over time: a controversial mechanism*

Since the beginning of the 20th century, both the American Cancer Society (ACS) in the United States and the *Ligue nationale contre le cancer* (LNCC, National Cancer League) in France have been campaigning for the early detection of cancers.

At the end of the 1930s, a clinical detection technique was developed that was carried out in the professional's office during a medical consultation, based on a visual examination and palpation of suspected nodules by the expert. The second systematized detection technique is self-palpation[3]. Twenty years later, clinical breast examinations and breast self-examination were joined by a third screening technique: mammography. Starting in the 1970s, this last technique is supposed to be a reliable tool for screening asymptomatic populations. In the decades that followed, it became an increasingly common medical practice without public consultation [BOI 03, MEN 07]. It was gynecologists, industrialists and private practitioners, particularly radiologists, who facilitated its diffusion [MEN 07]. It was not until the 1980s that mammography became an essential part of the detection system in France.

In France, the organized breast cancer screening program was launched in 2004. This program is based on specifications published in the government gazette of the French Republic (*Journal official de la République française*) of December 21, 2006[4], which define and frame its procedures, monitoring and evaluation. All women over the age of 50 and up to their 75th birthday – 9.5 million women in 2010 – are thus required to undergo a mammogram every two years, which is fully covered by health insurance. The stakes are high from a public health perspective. More than 22 million mammography screenings have been organized in this way. The five-year net survival rate for breast cancer was 86% for people diagnosed

3 "Breast self-examination or self-testing is a set of simple actions that, practiced every month after your period, allow you to get to know your breasts well, to detect any abnormality and to report it to your doctor." According to the site "*Cancer du sein, parlons-en—!*" https://www.cancerdusein.org/le-depistage/lauto-examen-des-seins.

4 Order of December 29, 2006 on cancer screening programs: https://www.legifrance.gouv.fr/afficheTexte.do;jsessionid=3FF7D9D2BFEB7FD55A29E2BFA395F60F.tpdila18v_2?cidTexte=JORFTEXT000000460656&dateTexte=&oldAction=rechJO&categorieLien=id&idJO=JORFCONT000000006642.

between 1989 and 2004[5]. In 2014, more than one out of two women participated in this screening program, or nearly 2,520,000 people according to the French National Cancer Institute *Institut national des cancers* (INCa). In addition to these figures, approximately 10–15% of women undergo screening mammograms at the request of their physician or on their own initiative, a practice known as spontaneous or opportunistic or individual screening (IS)[6]. Screening, whether individual or organized, is now present in the daily medical lives of women aged 50–74 years. The number of institutions and information and communication forums on primary and secondary prevention has increased.

For more than a century, both breast cancer experts and their official institutions have adhered to the principle of early diagnosis and treatment, which organizes the medico-centric standards of screening, but this hegemony is ever more contested [JUN 03]. Every screening program is open to debate and, for both the expert and the lay person, there may be many questions in terms of accuracy or safety, for example, how many people are likely to be false negatives?

What type of effective treatment is available to eradicate the symptoms of the disease detected? Are these treatments themselves safe? If the treatment appears to be risky, to what extent should it be imposed on people who may never have developed any symptoms? The examination of these questions is today reserved for the judgment of experts [MEN 07].

Organized screening was questioned long before it was definitively established nationwide. The end of the 1980s saw the first divergent opinions emerge, but it was in 2000 that the latent controversy really began, and it has continued to develop to this day. In turn, different researchers [JUN 04] and practitioners [BOI 04, VEN 07] affirm the usefulness of the breast cancer screening program through studies establishing its ineffectiveness, while others refute the opinions previously expressed, reaffirming this usefulness. Media coverage of these peer discussions reinforces the controversy, ultimately raising the benefit/risk ratio [DEL 16] associated with this early detection device. A militant movement, outside the medical and health framework, against screening has emerged largely in the United States [MEN 10], as well as in France, notably with the publication in 2011 of

5 http://www.e-cancer.fr/Professionnels-de-sante/Depistage-et-detection-precoce/Depistage-du-cancer-du-sein/Le-programme-de-depistage-organise#toc-le-d-pistage-organis-en-quelques-chiffres.

6 Health figures: http://invs.santepubliquefrance.fr//Espace-presse/Communiques-de-presse/2014/October-October-2014-Each-woman-screening-adapted-to-her-risk-level.

Rachel Campergue's *No Mammo: enquête sur le dépistage du cancer du sein*[7]. Since then, we have seen individual and collective initiatives in the same direction.

The citizen and public scientific consultation[8] conducted in France in 2016 brought about these points of discussion, as it is clear that the objectives set at the beginning of the organized screening program were struggling to be achieved. As the program grew more and more from one year to the next, it was only after four years of conducting the program at the national level that a stagnation in the participation rate[9] was observed. The rates recorded since 2008 have been around 50%, as the program was intended to be a scheme in which nearly 80% of the women concerned (aged 50–74 years) would participate. Even if there are measurable differences between territories and socio-economic groups, the figures are still far from the initial ambitions[10]. Moreover, the questioning of the mortality rate, an indicator used to measure changes in the system, does not argue in favor of the program. Indeed, it is difficult today to assert and prove that a possible decrease in mortality from breast cancer would be directly linked to the presence of a breast cancer screening program[11]. As previously mentioned, the report produced after this consultation[12] also points out the risks associated with screening in itself, which may lead to false positives or false negatives, over-diagnosis or over-medicalization, or to incurring certain risks related to radiotherapy.

At the end of this citizen and public consultation, the public authorities very recently, on April 21, 2017, pronounced new measures, notably on information processes, the integration of women over 25 years of age in an information and monitoring system, and the strengthening of the role of the general practitioner and the gynecologist in the information and awareness system.

These new measures, strongly encouraged by the INCa, seem to be moving towards individualized prevention rather than mass prevention, as has been the case

7 No Mammo(gram): survey on breast cancer screening.

8 http://www.concertation-depistage.fr/#donne-avis.

9 http://www.santepubliquefrance.fr/Actualites/Donnees-de-participation-au-programme-de-depistage-organise-du-cancer-du-sein-2015-2016.

10 http://invs.santepubliquefrance.fr/Dossiers-thematiques/Maladies-chroniques-et-traumatismes/Cancers/Evaluation-des-programmes-de-depistage-des-cancers/Evaluation-du-programme-de-depistage-du-cancer-du-sein/Indicateurs-d-evaluation/Taux-de-participation-au-programme-de-depistage-organise-du-cancer-du-sein-2015-2016.

11 This reflection is all the more necessary because in 2012 in France, nearly 48,800 new cases of breast cancer and 11,886 deaths were recorded.

12 To consult the final report resulting from the digital contributions: http://www.concertation-depistage.fr/wp-content/uploads/2016/10/concertations-screening-breast cancer-analysis-contributions-digital-june-2016.pdf.

until now. It remains to be seen, in a few years' time, how these measures will be implemented and how they will be perceived by both the population concerned and the health actors. The latter, as we will see in section 5.2.1.2, raise some questions about their multiplicity and the overlapping of their competences.

OVER-DIAGNOSIS. –

Over-diagnosis refers to the diagnosis of a problem that, had it not been found, would not have caused symptoms or death. In other words, it is the detection of a problem without any possible benefit to be gained from early treatment of the person concerned. Misdiagnosis and false positives are related but distinctly different concepts. Misdiagnosis is the incorrect identification of a problem, often owing to a lack of diagnostic specificity, such as attributing swelling and redness in the big toe to cellulite rather than gout. False positives occur when the initial results of a test used to investigate an abnormality, such as microcalcification observed in mammography, are positive, but the results of a follow-up test (such as a biopsy) do not reveal any pathology.

OVERMEDICALIZATION –

"The notion of overmedicalization refers to medical practices that have not been validated in terms of their benefits to patients and are potentially harmful and therefore unnecessarily costly" [HAN 16]. This could be related to the permanent expansion of information about treatments, particularly via the Web, the promotion of diseases, the inadequate management of diagnostic uncertainty, conflicts of interest or the lack of commitment of physicians and patients to a shared decision-making process [HAN 16].

5.2.1.2. *The multiplicity of actors in prevention: intertwined skills*

There is a plurality of actors, and therefore of logics and interests, in the field of prevention: users, doctors, associations, pharmaceutical companies, local authorities, the State and so on. Multiple interactions between these actors create a real complexity in decision-making in the field of prevention. In France, competences in the field of prevention are shared between the State and local authorities, which does not contribute to the comprehensibility of the system as a whole. In addition to the relevant departments of the Ministry of Health, many other players (specialized bodies, public or para-public organizations) are involved in the prevention system. Since 1992, a series of agencies and autonomous public establishments have been created to deal with the sectoral aspects of public health policy[13]. In addition to this,

13 The *Agence française de sécurité sanitaire des produits de santé* (AFSSAPS, French Agency for the Safety of Health Products), the *Haut Comité de santé publique* (High Public Health Committee), which is responsible for defining risks and prevention objectives, the *Institut national de veille sanitaire* (INVS, National Institute for Public Health Surveillance),

institutional representation of users has emerged in France since the 1996 Juppé ordinances. The public authorities have conferred institutional legitimacy on patient, consumer and family associations [DEM 00].

The multiplication of institutions could lead to tangled skills, lack of synergy or coordination, as well as to social inequalities in access to prevention awareness information and/or organized screening. The INCa[14] report, commissioned by the French National Health Agency to evaluate and reorganize the breast cancer prevention screening system, highlights the heterogeneity of these structures in terms of the expected results and the information systems used.

In addition to the institutional players in prevention, it should be noted that the number of companies committed to raising awareness against breast cancer has continued to grow over the years. Estée Lauder, Avon, Komen, the company Zeneca Pharmaceutical, producer of tamoxifen, the world's best-selling breast cancer drug, as well as other commercial and non-commercial organizations, participate in several events and activities during the month of October. This awareness-raising operation is known in France as "Pink October". In October 1994, the Estée Lauder Group, in association with *Marie France* magazine, created the awareness campaign entitled "*Le cancer du sein, parlons-en*" (Breast cancer, let's talk about it). At the same time, movements against the exploitation of this cause by industrialists have emerged, such as the "Think before you pink" movement launched in 2002 to raise awareness among Americans about what they call "pink washing". In 2016, the League Against Cancer created a "Stop pink washing" charter[15] to raise awareness among its employees against the mercantile and opportunistic excesses of this event.

Undeniably, breast cancer prevention evolves in a context of strategic sociopolitical and medical-health uncertainty owing to the questioning of its normative ideology, a non-individualized and scientifically contrasted system, and a set of intertwined actors and skills that struggle to achieve their "objectives". Moreover, it is difficult to grasp these uncertainties without reflecting on individual behaviors in the face of health risks and on their perceptions and practices within this uncertain prevention context. In organizing this reflection, the contribution of the social and human sciences and the information and communication sciences, in

---

the *Comité technique national de prévention* (National Prevention Technical Committee), *Institut national de prévention et d'éducation pour la santé* (INPES, National Institute for Prevention and Education for Health) and others all have a role to play.

14 Evolution of the organization of the cancer screening system/referral response: http://www.senologie.com/wp-content/uploads/2016/12/evolution-de-l-organisation-of-the-cancer-screening-device_20161207.pdf.

15 Available at: http://www.liguecancer44.fr/actualite/stop-au-pinkwashing/ (accessed October 6, 2017).

particular, seems undeniable. Communication campaigns and organized screening systems are becoming increasingly important. They arouse both hope and fear, criticism and contentment. We are all concerned by this public health issue, so the reactions are marked by the experiences of each and every one of us. As a result, the human and social sciences, and more particularly the information and communication sciences, come to grasp the complexity of exchanges and contexts. They make it possible to provide a theoretical and methodological reference framework for the perception and individual and collective representations of breast cancer prevention systems.

5.3. Methodological choices for the analysis of an online exchange space

Health research on the Internet has multiplied over the last 15 years with the development of Internet and mobile technology use by the population and caregivers. A field of studies has been established, which is referred to as e-health studies [KIV 13]. Whether quantitative or qualitative, studies in the human and social sciences in the field of health on the Internet offer new opportunities to the researcher [THO 16]. This study allowed us to follow up on our corpus for two years (2015/2016), not to be restricted to a geographical area (anyone interested in the subject could take part), to go and find the women affected by the screening where they were (the choice of the exchange space), to decide whether to be anonymous or not (anonymity allowing participants to intervene freely), to be able to be in contact with participants in order to complete this study (interview, focus group, etc.) and so on. We collect text, video and image data. We are also interested in digital traces, such as emoticons on Facebook and sharing. We are also collecting the number of messages, contributions, *likes,* shares, subscribers and so on.

5.3.1. *Boundaries of the field: study by the Facebook group "Cancer du sein, parlons-en" (Breast cancer, let's talk about it)*

After a phase of identification and exploration of different spaces of exchange around breast cancer and its prevention, it seemed important to us to delimit our study space. We decided to analyze the Facebook exchange group "*Cancer du sein, parlons-en*"[16] for different reasons; first of all because of its relevance to the topic under study, the large number of contributions in relation to the other spaces

16 Since our study, the association and the Facebook page have changed their name to "*Le cancer du sein, parlons-en parler!*". We have kept the name of the page at the time of the research here.

identified and, finally, the link that the editorial choices of this space could have with the founder of this space, which is the Estée Lauder group [OMR 16].

Founded in 1946 in New York City, the Estée Lauder company, specializing in cosmetic products, is rapidly internationalizing and diversifying its product line. Starting in 1992, the family business, at the initiative of Evelyn H. Lauder, vice-president of the worldwide Estée Lauder Group, co-created the Pink Ribbon with *Self Magazine,* which has become the single largest campaign against breast cancer. The following year, in 1993, the company created the Breast Cancer Research Foundation (BCRF) in the United States to support innovation in clinical and genetic research. In October 1994, the Estée Lauder France cosmetics group joined forces with *Marie Claire* magazine to found the association "*Le cancer du sein, parlons-en–!*" This association is omnipresent on socio-digital dispositives (Facebook, Twitter, message boards).

In this study, we are interested in one of its features: the association's Facebook page, "*Cancer du sein, parlons-en*"[17]. We analyzed the content of this page during the "Pink October" event. This digital page was created in 2009, and it is followed today by 724,963 people[18]. Our corpus is limited to the messages published by the association during the months of October 2015/2016, that is, 80 topics and an average of 50 comments per topic, comprising a corpus of about 4,000 texts.

It should be noted that the "organization of exchanges" [AKR 09] on "*Cancer du sein, parlons-en*" is distinguished by the very characteristics of the social–digital network Facebook. The contents are initiated entirely by the association's community manager; nevertheless, these contents are often relayed and not produced.

In terms of interaction, the initial content elicits on average hundreds of "likes" and "shares" and about 50 comments. Threads are varied and may not be related to the original topic. The majority of participants are female, and either following treatment, in remission or close to a patient[19]. Most caregivers log in with their Facebook account and their own identity.

---

17 This analysis is part of a more global study on the social–medical mechanisms of breast cancer prevention (field observation, interviews and analysis of the contents of an RSN corpus concerned by this issue). Study conducted during the "Pink October" event from October 1 to 31, 2015/2016/2017.

18 Cancerduseinparlonsen.com is one of the socio-digital devices on breast cancer identified for our study as the most frequently visited and most active in terms of user participation.

19 Breast cancer in men is rare. Less than 1% of all breast cancers affect men. In our corpus, we found only one testimonial from a male patient with breast cancer.

COMMUNITY MANAGERS/COMMUNITY MANAGEMENT. –

The community manager (CM) is the one who, within an organization, manages the community link between a certain number of actors. Previously, this link was correlated to geographical location since members shared a community and purpose, as is the case for associations. With the advent of digital social networks, we talk more about communities of interest, since what makes the link is then based on tastes, practices, interests, passions, claimed or at least assumed membership, etc. [STE 11]. It is a profession that is emerging and under construction. However, we can still uncover several CM models: "the supporter, the animator, the developer and the watchman" [STE 11]. These are professional practices that are the most recurrent in this type of profession.

5.3.2. *Online non-participant observation*

For this phase of the study, we decided to conduct non-participant observations. Indeed, we found it sensitive and intrusive to contribute to the group's discussions even though this could be done in a more focused manner in a later phase of the study. In the health field, the study of online exchange spaces raises particular ethical issues related to the sensitivity of the practices and the nature of the material. The boundary between private and public in this field is complex. The perception that participants have of the private or public nature of the exchange space in which they participate is therefore an important issue. People who are ill or who have ill relatives and who rely on anonymity to participate in these forums could suffer from the intrusion of a researcher in their community if the publication of research results made it possible to identify the participants or discussion spaces [THO 12b]. We therefore engaged in an invisible ethnography [KIT 07], without declaring our presence and without potentially impacting the results of our research.

In order not to be overwhelmed by the amount of data and without restricting our field of observation too much, we relied on an observation grid. This was constructed thanks to the first exploratory observations of the exchange space, takes up the elements of uncertainty around prevention identified in the literature and obviously remains open to incorporate emerging elements of observation.

The themes that we initially identified for these observations concerned:

– the type of prevention (primary, secondary, tertiary);

– the editor of the message, the reference to the history and evolution of prevention;

– the type of discourse and its references, perceptions and practices related to the prevention discourse;

– participant profiles, and finally, we tried to identify what the following words or their synonyms related to: trust, mistrust, risk, uncertainty.

5.4. Results of ethnographic observation and lexicometric analysis

Content analysis using NVivo software allowed us to confirm one of our first online observation results. Indeed, this breast cancer prevention space revealed activities characteristic of online social [GAU 12] or emotional support [THO 12a]. Online social support varies according to the media used, and does not always resemble social support between close friends and family (no prior closeness) or a discussion group (the institution is not necessarily the originator and there is not necessarily any encouragement). However, the interest here is in understanding the benefits associated with different levels of participation [CHE 19].

The lexicometric analysis we conducted confirms the concealment of a lexicographical field: prevention and screening. On the other hand, we found expressions that fall within the register of emotional support, informative contribution or tangible support (see the word cloud in Figure 5.1). Indeed, in a context of uncertainty, as described above, this exchange space initially dedicated to prevention and awareness of early detection becomes a social support mechanism generating, not without interest for its publishers, an abundance of content.

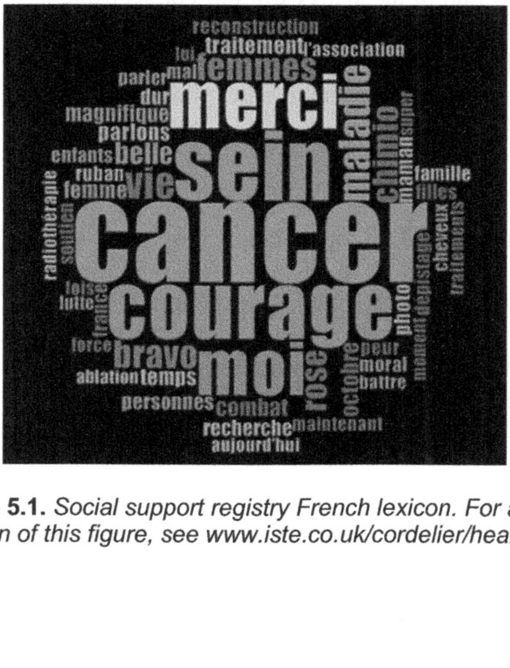

Figure 5.1. *Social support registry French lexicon. For a color version of this figure, see www.iste.co.uk/cordelier/health.zip*

ONLINE SOCIAL SUPPORT. –

Researchers of online social support use the definitions and typology of traditional social support [BAR 94, WAL 02], as reported in Gauducheau's literature review [GAU 12] devoted to this subject. Indeed, "social support is the exchange of messages that convey emotions or information to help reduce uncertainty or stress, and that directly or indirectly signal to the person that they are valued and cared for" [GAU 12, p. 96]. We also find the same typology of online social support: informational, emotional, evaluative and tangible. In this approach, we can also see the presence of the principle of "caregiver therapy". This reveals the *empowerment* effect of offering support. This is particularly the case with the patient's expertise. In this context, counseling offers a status to the patient close to that of the expert. A final form of support is present: that of social comparison highlights the positive and negative impacts of comparing one's personal situation with the experiences of others facing a similar problem. The social compensation/enhancement model was used to understand the relationship between access to offline support and use of online support [CHE 19].

5.4.1. *The emotional support registry*

Emotional support tends to describe the provision of comfort, friendship, love or sympathy [BAR 02]. Lexicometric analysis (frequency and conditions of use of words in the corpus analyzed) revealed a high rate of the following occurrences: courage, bravo, thank you, moral, struggle, fight, fear, strength, magic, photo and so on [BAR 02]. We also find in the analysis of our corpus expressions such as: it's going to be okay, hope, you have to live, you are not alone, fight and so on. One of the particularities of this lexicon of emotional support lies in the presence of a warlike vocabulary. It is a "war" against the disease, which would imply cohesion between the different actors.

PRIMARY, SECONDARY AND TERTIARY PREVENTION MESSAGES. –

According to the HALDE, "prevention consists of avoiding the appearance, development or aggravation of diseases or disabilities; a distinction is usually made between primary prevention, which acts upstream of the disease (e.g. vaccination and action on risk factors), secondary prevention, which acts at an early stage in its evolution (screening), and tertiary prevention, which acts on complications and the risk of recurrence"[20] (see the definition of "prevention" in section 5.2).

20 https://www.has-sante.fr/jcms/c_410178/fr/prevention.

Primary prevention messages concerning risk factors (diet, sports activity, lifestyle) are very rare (two out of 40 during the month of October). They are part of the impersonal system of prevention and the individual responsibility for health. This position most often presents itself in terms of lifestyle choices and encourages, for example, exercising, eating healthily and giving up smoking as much as it does adhering to the principles of early detection. We have found that these messages elicit very little interaction but a lot of sharing. If interactions are infrequent, they are often criticized by people with breast cancer. Sharing is thus a symbol of content that is recognized as useful. This content is valued because, for example, it is scientifically proven. However, when there are interactions, they are confronted with the experiences and personal stories of people with breast cancer. It is then that the posts can be experienced as a judgment on life choices and reasons for the illness. Prevention is experienced, for some, as a judgment and as a negative element.

The secondary prevention messages here concern early detection and visual support in the form of posters or videos. Interactions around these messages are only between patients; the public affected by screenings does not participate. The initial prevention message is often hijacked into accounts of experiences. The interactions here focus on experiences of mammography screening and self-testing. Patients in remission often see themselves here as spokespersons for the benefits of screening: "If I had not been screened, it would have become very serious [...]." Other testimonials highlight or question the skills of the radiologist and the attending physician in diagnosing the pathology.

Tertiary prevention messages, concerning the social and professional reintegration of the patient, most often take the form of book publications, blogs, video reports or media testimonies of patients in remission, as shown in the example below:

> Breast cancer: two women from Nîmes testify. Martine Gayraud and Martine Munoz both fought the disease. As part of Pink October, the month that raises awareness about breast cancer prevention, they share their experiences... On midilibre.fr.

These testimonials encourage encouragement and interaction on the representation of self and body in relation to the pre-disease: "I fought and struggled, I momentarily won. But every day, I feel like shouting "give me back my life as it was before" (post of October 16, 2016); "my left breast has been removed, I find my body pretty as it is now, my scar is very beautiful, I live with it very well, my other half too, and if my right breast was affected in turn I would not hesitate to have it removed..." (published October 11, 2016).

We can also mention the interactions following one of the two key moments in the "Pink October" period that are the subject of an advertisement. This is the Estée Lauder Pink Ribbon Photo Award. Indeed, this event generates a lot of interaction, especially from the general public: "Strength, Faith, Courage! Never lose hope! [...]"; "I support all the sick because no one is safe from this..."; "great photo, we must clench our fists, my ladies, have faith in courage, be strong with you until you win". We also find reactions to the photograph presented: "[...] magnificent photo that breathes life [heart]"; "very nice photo [...]" (excerpts from posts of October 4, 2016).

The interactions are not often related to the content of the initial message and are rather, as is often the case in digital health exchange dispositives, oriented towards life stories [STA 12], with many exchanges that are more of an emotional and social support nature. In our study, for each type of prevention, the interactions essentially concern life stories that retrace the therapeutic (diagnosis, treatment, surgery, medical follow-up) and social (relationship with the doctor and the medical profession, the patient's family and friends, the importance of psychological support) pathways. In these interactions, we note words that appear quite frequently in the discourse (it's going to be okay, hope, you have to live, you are not alone, courage, fight, strength, fight, etc.) and the relationships that are created between practitioners (adding to the list of Facebook friends, nominative requests for news).

5.4.2. *Informational input and tangible support*

The informational input could be an aid to problem solving, decision-making and judgment regarding a medical diagnosis, treatment process or screening, and so on. The most common words that fall under this heading are: treatment, chemo, radiotherapy, ablation and reconstruction. This support is not only about medical information or opinion. Aesthetics, social environment, sexuality or post-cancer life can be the subject of these informational exchanges.

Finally, even if material support is not identified as such in this study, tangible support can manifest itself in the interpersonal links that are created between participants (addition to the Facebook friends list, nominative requests for news, invitation to a conference or training session on taking care of one's body, etc.). Obviously, these social support activities are not distinct, or sequential; we may find in the same message a person who reacts emotionally to a photo (Photo Awards) by referring to his or her problem (a recurrence, or non-acceptance of a body change), which triggers messages of emotional support, encouragement or the story of an experience that contains information and advice.

The invisible links that form in these exchange spaces progressively become strong links of transmission of knowledge from personal experiences. This knowledge can be at the origin of a decision-making process or of a judgment regarding a health program. Confidence is acquired not through medical and scientific information provided by health actors, but through interpersonal exchanges that can reduce or accentuate both types of uncertainty: strategic and final adjustment. The informational contribution in these interactions, based on the individual experience of patients or screened individuals, is therefore essential in the context in which breast cancer screening is evolving in France. In fact, despite the info-communication systems deployed by public players, notably the INCa, only 52% of women in France between 50 and 75 years of age responded to the screening organized in 2017–2018. This participation rate, in addition to being below the 2006 European benchmark, which recommends a participation rate of 70% or more for the target population, has been declining since 2011. This decrease could be explained by the controversy over the benefit–risk of screening as explained above, as well as by the lack of awareness or rejection of info-communication dispositives from public actors aimed at the people concerned by breast cancer screening. This observation is confirmed by the study we are currently conducting among general practitioners in Haute-Garonne, France. Indeed, in the absence of a consultation dedicated to screening, few patients come to their doctor for advice. If the doctor does bring up the subject, the time constraint does not allow her or him to answer all the patient's questions and she or he chooses to refer her to public information spaces or recognized medical–technical websites. Consulted or not, these sources of information lack individualization in the discourse and often do not allow exchanges with peers. This is how discussion groups such as "*Le cancer du sein, parlons-en*" become information and communication tools for the prevention of breast cancer, characterized by interpersonal exchanges between patients and/or the people concerned by screening. These new informational systems are becoming a significant issue that public players in the field of prevention must take into consideration in their communication policy.

Finally, it should be pointed out that the intervention of community managers is very rare in the context of social support. This can be explained by the difficulty of moderating or refocusing exchanges. Moderating intimate, personal content can end an exchange and, in particular, prevent the person interacting with the Facebook page. It can also alter the trust between the platform and the participants. Here, we are faced with hypotheses, and we should complete our research with interviews with participants and community managers to confirm or refute our statements.

In addition, Estée Lauder, as mentioned in section 5.3.1, is doubly present on social–digital networks: through its own commercial platforms (Facebook, Instagram, Pinterest, Twitter, YouTube channel) and through the "*Cancer du sein, parlons-en!*" association, which is itself omnipresent on socio-digital devices

(Facebook, Twitter, message boards). The company is showing itself to be a good corporate citizen. The number of visitors to this exchange space that we have studied here, the topics discussed and the lack of a policy to refocus interactions confirm the use of content marketing techniques and the attention economy of online platforms for exchanges on health. The mobilization of socio-digital networks by Estée Lauder to serve its social and civic responsibility in the fight against breast cancer seems obvious to us and arouses our interest as a researcher in information and communication sciences. Is this not what we are looking for: to generate “emotional” content to serve the institutionalization of CSR (corporate social responsibility) communication? The official prevention discourse, on the other hand, is minimized because it generates very few reactions (attention) and content (contribution) [OMR 16].

5.5. Conclusion

The cultural, historical and organizational context of breast cancer prevention reveals a crisis of confidence and two types of uncertainties: “strategic uncertainties” concerning the choices related to the prevention program and “final adjustment uncertainties” concerning the judgment of this program and the screening decisions made by the population concerned. Our approach focused on what people who interact on social–digital networks think about prevention campaigns and their online info-communication practices.

Based on Lucien Karpik’s analysis grid [KAR 07], on the trust mechanisms of the users of a service, carrying out content analysis (October 2015 and 2016) of the Facebook page of a breast cancer association allowed us to identify two trust mechanisms: an interpersonal mechanism, based on social support, and an impersonal medico-technical mechanism, based on standards, certification or simply trust in the skills of health professionals [KAP 08] and institutional discourse [OMR 18]. Even if we do not report on the latter system here, it is worth noting that prevention discourse in France is mainly based on incentives and comes from institutions, whether public or associative, as explained above. The discourses analyzed on the digital social network studied reveal compliance or rejection practices on the part of the population concerned. The interactions provoked by these prevention discourses essentially belong to the emotional register. In addition to the emergence and proliferation of the discourse of the new actors in prevention, such as cancer patients, those in remission or their friends and family, we note that the discourse on the medico-technical promise and individual responsibility is flawed.

In a context of uncertainty, the interpersonal dispositives of trust through social support, knowledge sharing and life stories are increasingly important. They are indicative of shared online representations, particularly those related to uncertainties about health promotion in general and breast cancer prevention in particular. Indeed, medical information on social networks symbolizes the advent of users who question the boundaries of expertise and who value lay expertise based on experiential knowledge [FRA 05, PAG 14]. Faced with a medical profession and public institutions that evoke illness in different ways, we have thus observed that, for the individual, it is relationships with others that are at the heart of discourse, and their lifestyle, their social identity and their experiences. Trust seems to us to be co-constructed in a process rooted in individual realities and social support between people affected by breast cancer. At the same time, public authorities are still struggling to master prevention campaigns and communications relating to health crises in general [OLL 15] (the latest in progress concerns the Levothyrox case). It seems to us that these communication strategies are far from being adapted to the online info-communication practices of the population concerned (social links, sharing of experiences, life stories, mediation, etc.); however, these strategies offer new perspectives for prevention and health promotion in general [REN 12]. Faced with a desire to re-singularize prevention (construction of meaning *in situ,* comparison and individualization of situations, individualization of the information process and the use of prevention dispositives), public and official players in breast cancer prevention and screening should rethink their communication and health promotion strategy. This is a communication dispositive involving the population concerned, beyond the medical–technical discourse or the individual responsibility of the population concerned.

5.6. References

[AKR 09] AKRICH M., MEADEL C., “Les échanges entre patients sur l’Internet”, *La Presse médicale*, no. 38, pp. 1484–1490, 2009.

[AKR 12] AKRICH M., RABEHARISOA V., “L’expertise profane dans les associations de patients, un outil de démocratie sanitaire”, *Santé Publique*, vol. 24, pp. 69–74, 2012.

[BAR 94] BARNES M.K., DUCK S., “Everyday communicative contexts for social support”, in BURLESON B. (ed.), *Communication of Social Support: Messages, Interactions, Relationships and Community*, Sage Publications, Thousand Oaks, 1994.

[BAR 02] BARRERA M., “Do internet-based support interventions change perceptions of social support? An experimental trial of approaches for supporting diabetes self-management”, *American Journal of Community Psychology*, vol. 30, no. 5, pp. 637–654, 2002.

[BAR 07] BARREAU B., “La communication vers les femmes et leur information”, in SERADOUR B. (ed.), *Le dépistage du cancer du sein : un enjeu de santé publique*, Springer Science & Business Media, Berlin, 2007.

[BAR 09] BARBARA L., *From Pink to Green: Disease Prevention and the Environmental Breast Cancer Movement*, Rutgers University Press, New Brunswick, 2009.

[BAR 14] BARTHE Y., CALLON M., LASCOUMES P., *Agir dans un monde incertain. Essai sur la démocratie technique*, Le Seuil, Paris, 2014.

[BEN 11] BENDER L.-J., JIMENEZ-MARROQUIN M.-C., JADAD R., "Seeking support on Facebook: A content analysis of breast cancer groups", *J. Med. Internet Res.*, vol. 13, no. 1, 2011.

[BER 03] BERTOLOTTO F., JOUBERT M., LEROUX M. *et al.*, "Facteurs sociaux de l'absence de participation aux campagnes de dépistage de masse du cancer du sein", *Bull. épidémiol. hebd.*, 2003.

[BOI 04] BOISSONNAT V., "Fausses évidences et vrais dilemmes en santé publique : le dépistage radiologique des cancers du sein", *Santé Publique*, vol. 16, no. 1, pp. 9–20, 2004.

[CAL 04] CALVEZ M., *La prévention du sida : les sciences sociales et la définition des risques*, Presses Universitaires de Rennes, Rennes, 2004.

[CHE 19] CHERBA M., THOËR C., TURBIDE O. *et al.*, "Le soutien social en ligne comme mode d'intervention psychosociale : revue de littérature, pistes de recherche et recommandations pour les intervenants", *Santé Publique*, vol. 31, no. 1, pp. 83–92, 2019.

[COU 09] COURBET D., BERNARD F., JOULE R.-V. *et al.*, "Communication numérique engageante et protection de l'environnement : effets immédiats et différés sur les comportements, l'attitude et la mémorisation", *3ème Colloque international psychologie sociale et communication*, Tarbes, France, 22–24 June 2009.

[COU 13] COURBET D., FOURQUET-COURBET M.-P., BERNARD F. *et al.*, "Communication persuasive et communication engageante pour la santé. Favoriser des comportements sains avec les médias, Internet et les serious games", in BLANC N. (ed.), *Publicité et santé : des liaisons dangereuses ? Le point de vue de la psychologie*, In Press, Paris, 2013.

[DOL 09] DOLBEAULT S., BLAY J.Y., EISINGER F. *et al.*, "Cancers, cultures et pratiques de soins. Freins et motivations au dépistage des cancers du sein : quels profils typologiques ? Résultats issus de l'enquête ÉDIFICE. XXVème Congrès de la SFPO", *Psycho-oncologie*, vol. 3, no. 1, pp. 60–62, 2009.

[DUP 07] DUPORT N., ANCELLE-PARK R., BOUSSAC-ZAREBSKA M. *et al.*, Facteurs d'adhésion au dépistage organisé du cancer du sein : étude FADO-sein, Institut de veille sanitaire, Saint-Maurice, 2007.

[FRA 12] FRANCEQUIN G., *Cancer du sein : une féminité à reconstruire*, Érès, Toulouse, 2012.

[GAU 12] GAUDUCHEAU N., "Internet et le soutien social", in THOËR C., LEVY J.J. (eds), *Internet et santé, usages, acteurs et appropriations*, Presses de l'Université du Québec, Quebec, 2012.

[GAU 19] GAUDEMET A., "Qu'est-ce que la compliance ?", *Commentaire*, vol. 1, no. 165, pp. 109–114, 2019.

[GIO 12] GIORDANO L., VON KARSA L., TOMATIS M. *et al.*, "Mammographic screening programmes in Europe: Organization, coverage and participation", *Journal of Medical Screening*, vol. 19, no. 1, pp. 72–82, 2012.

[GOR 09] GORZA M., SALINES E., DANZON A. *et al.*, Programme de dépistage du cancer du sein en France : résultats 2006, Institut de veille sanitaire, Paris, 2009.

[HAN 16] HANSLIK T., FLAHAULT A., "La surmédicalisation : quand trop de médecine nuit à la santé", *La revue de médecine interne*, vol. 37, no. 3, pp. 201–205, 2016.

[HER 73] HERZLICH C., *Health and Illness: A Social Psychological Analysis*, vol. 5, Academic Press, London, 1973.

[INC 13] INCA, Bénéfices et limites du programme de dépistage organisé du cancer du sein. Quels éléments en 2013 ? Available at: www.e-cancer.fr/.../Benefices-limites-du-programme-de-depistage-cancer-sein2013.p, 2013.

[JUN 03] JUNOD B., MASSE R., "Dépistage du cancer du sein et médicalisation de la santé publique", *Santé Publique*, vol. 15, no. 2, pp. 125–129, 2003.

[JUN 04] JUNOD B., MASSE R., QUELIER C., "Cancer du sein : danger des certitudes prétendues", *Santé Publique*, vol. 16, no. 1, pp. 21–26, 2004.

[KAL 15] KALECINSKI J., REGNIER-DENOIS V., OUEDRAOGO S. *et al.*, "Dépistage organisé ou individuel du cancer du sein ? Attitudes et représentations des femmes", *Santé Publique*, vol. 27, no. 2, pp. 213–220, 2015.

[KAR 07] KARPIK L., *L'économie des singularités*, Gallimard, Paris, 2007.

[KHA 14] KHAYAT D., *Prévenir le cancer, ça dépend aussi de vous*, Odile Jacob, Paris, 2014.

[KIV 16] KIVITS J., *Les recherches qualitatives en santé*, Armand Collin, Paris, 2016.

[LOU 04] LOUBIERE S., PARENT A., TALLON J.-M., "L'économie de la prévention : enjeux et problématiques", *Revue économique*, pp. 831–847, 2004.

[MAR 10a] MARCHIOLI A., La communication d'action et d'utilité sociétales : étude de la production et de la réception de la communication médiatique préventive du sida, Perspectives ouvertes par la communication engageante, Information and Communication Sciences, PhD Thesis, Aix-Marseille Université, Marseille, 2010.

[MAR 10b] MARCHIOLI A., COURBET D., "Communication de santé publique et prévention du sida. Une expérimentation sur l'influence de mini-actes engageants via Internet", *Hermès, La Revue*, vol. 3, no. 58, pp. 167–174, 2010.

[MEA 14] MEADLE C., "Partager ma propre opinion", *Le Temps des médias*, no. 23, pp. 128–140, 2014.

[MEN 06] MENORET M., "Prévention du cancer du sein : cachez ce politique que je ne saurais voir", *Nouvelles questions féministes*, vol. 25, pp. 32–47, 2006.

[MEN 07a] MENORET M., "Incertitude médicale et rhétorique statistique en cancérologie", *Sciences sociales et santé*, vol. 25, no. 1, pp. 33–54, 2007.

[MEN 07b] MENORET M., "Le risque de cancer du sein en France : un mode unique de prévention", *Sociologie et sociétés*, vol. 39, no. 1, pp. 145–160, 2007.

[MEN 10] MENORET M., "Objets ici, actrices là-bas. Les patientes françaises, passagères clandestines d'un mouvement social du cancer du sein", *Pratiques*, no. 49, pp. 32–36, 2010.

[MIG 18] MIGNOT P., OMRANE D., "Préventions des cancers du sein : ce que la controverse fait à l'action publique ?" *Les enjeux de l'information et de la communication*, Supplement A, 2018.

[OLL 15] OLLIVIER-YANIV C., "La communication publique sanitaire à l'épreuve des controverses", *Hermès, La Revue*, vol. 73, no. 3, pp. 69–80, 2015.

[OMR 16] OMRANE D., "Médiation numérique de la responsabilité sociale d'entreprise : prévention contre le cancer du sein", *Revue française des sciences de l'information et de la communication*, no. 9, 2016.

[OMR 18] OMRANE D., MIGNOT P., "Communications de la prévention : confiance et légitimité en co-construction", in PAGANELLI C. (ed.), *Confidence and Legitimacy in Health Information and Communication*, ISTE Ltd, London and John Wiley & Sons, New York, 2018.

[OUE 15] OUEDRAOGO S., DABAKUYO-YONLI T.S., ROUSSOT A. *et al.*, "Dépistage du cancer du sein dans treize départements français", *Bulletin du Cancer*, vol. 102, no. 2, pp. 126–138, 2015.

[PAG 12] PAGANELLI C., Une approche info-communicationnelle des activités informationnelles en contexte de travail : acteurs, pratiques et logiques sociales, PhD Thesis, Université de Grenoble, Grenoble, 2012.

[PAG 14] PAGANELLI C., CLAVIER V., "S'informer via des médias sociaux de santé : quelle place pour les experts ?", *Le Temps des médias*, no. 2, pp. 141–143, 2014.

[PAI 07] PAILLIART I., STRAPPAZZON G., "Les paradoxes de la prévention des cancers : publicisation et privatisation", *Questions de communication*, pp. 17–31, 2007.

[PER 09] PERETTI-WATEL P., MOATTI J.-P., *Le principe de prévention*, Le Seuil, Paris, 2009.

[POR 10] PORNET C., DEJARDIN O., MORLAIS F. *et al.*, "Socioeconomic and healthcare supply statistical determinants of compliance to mammography screening programs: A multilevel analysis in calvados, France", *Cancer Epidemiology*, vol. 34, no. 3, pp. 309–315, 2010.

[QUE 01] QUERE L., "La structure cognitive et normative de la confiance", *Réseaux*, no. 4, pp. 125–152, 2001.

[QUE 05] QUERE L., "Les 'dispositifs de confiance' dans l'espace public", *Réseaux*, vol. 4, no. 132, pp. 185–217, 2005.

[REN 11] RENAUD L., "Internet et la promotion de la santé", in THOËR C., LEVY J.J. (eds), *Internet et santé, usages, acteurs et appropriations*, Presses de l'Université du Québec, Quebec, 2011.

[ROM 13] ROMEYER R., MOKTEFI A., "Pour une approche interdisciplinaire de la prévention", *Communication & Langages*, pp. 33–47, 2013.

[RUS 06] RUSSEL H., "Communautés et réseaux de confiance", in OGIEN A., QUERE L. (eds), *Les Moments de la confiance*, Economica, Paris, 2006.

[SAO 09] SAOUT C., "La crise de confiance dans le système de santé", *Les Tribunes de la santé*, no. 1, pp. 119–132, 2009.

[SIM 00] SIMPSON C., "Controversies in breast cancer prevention", in POTTS L. (ed.), *Ideologies of Breast Cancer, Feminist Perspectives*, St. Martin Press, New York, 2000.

[STE 11] STENGER T., COUTANT A., "Community management et community managers : Cheval de Troie marketing pour le web social ?", *Web social, communautés virtuelles et consommation*, vol. 140, 2011.

[SWE 14] SWEENEY E., "The individualization of risk and responsibility in breast cancer prevention education campaigns", *Policy Futures in Education*, vol. 12, no. 7, pp. 945–960, 2014.

[TES 13] TESCH R., *Qualitative Types: Analysis Typ.*, Routledge, London, 2013.

[THO 12a] THOËR C., "Les espaces d'échange en ligne consacrés à la santé : de nouvelles médiations de l'information santé", in THOËR C., LEVY J.J. (eds), *Internet et santé, usages, acteurs et appropriations, collection santé et société*, Presses de l'Université du Québec, Quebec, 2012.

[THO 12b] THOËR C., MILLERAND F., MYLES D. *et al.*, "Enjeux éthiques de la recherche sur les forums Internet portant sur l'utilisation des médicaments à des fins non médicales", *Communiquer*, no. 7, pp. 1–22, 2012.

[THO 14] THOËR C., LEVY J.J., *Internet et santé, usages, acteurs et appropriations*, Presses de l'Université du Québec, Quebec, 2014.

[THO 16] THOËR C., MILLERAND F., "Internet comme terrain d'investigation et mode de collecte des données qualitatives en santé", in KIVITS J. (ed.), *Les recherches qualitatives en santé*, Armand Collin, Paris, 2016.

[VER 07] VERNET A., HENRY F., "Prévention du cancer du sein et facteurs psychosociaux", *Le Journal des psychologues*, vol. 4, no. 247, pp. 54–57, 2007.

[WAL 02] WALTHER J.B., BOYD S., "Attraction to computer-mediated social support", in LIN C.A., ATKIN D. (eds), *Communication Technology and Society: Audience Adoption and Uses*, Hampton Press, Cresskill, 2002.

PART 3

Rethinking Health Expertise in Light of the Social Web

6

The Expert Patient in the Digital Age: Between Myth and Reality

6.1. Introduction

The idea that patients should be at the center of the healthcare system is a consensus throughout the world [BAS 10, POM 15] (*Plan santé 2022*, France's 2022 health plan). It emerged in the 1980s and 1990s with the questioning of the authority of health professionals and of the appropriateness of health policies (HIV, asbestos, contaminated blood, etc.). However, while in some English-speaking countries patient-centrality became effective in the 1990s, it is only since 2002 that in France we have seen the implementation of a legal and administrative apparatus around patients to ensure their place, with the Kouchner law (2002), the 2009 law on hospitals and the law on the modernization of the healthcare system of January 28, 2016. Since the turn of the 2000s, following the emergence of vocal associations, particularly of AIDS patients, patients have been recognized as having a form of expertise in their ability to search for and produce information, in their mastery of their pathology and in their experience of the disease. This slow recognition of the patient's expertise will crystallize in the figure of the expert patient. The expert patient is embodied in the form of patients who agree to help other patients to live better and to better understand their disease.

The aim of this chapter is to understand the emergence of expert patients in the digital age, first through a literature review and then through a survey of several patients. How did we move from paternalistic, self-centered medicine to participatory medicine sharing skills between health professionals and non-professionals? What is

---

Chapter written by Hélène ROMEYER.

the role and place of the digitization of the healthcare sector and the development of digital patient information practices?

To achieve this objective, we have made use of several of our previous works on online health information and the role of information and communication technologies (ICT) in the field of health, with analysis of discussion forums, in particular the place and role of life narratives and testimonials, questions and interviews with Internet users participating in online health forums. This work was supplemented by 10 interviews with expert patients. The panel of expert patients interviewed reveals an average age of 52.8 years; 71% of them are rural and therefore 29% of them urban; 42.8% are unemployed (retired or disabled), 28.6% are self-employed, 14.5% are engaged in a social activity and 14.1% are employed in the private sector.

The worked hypothesis is that expert patients are often seasoned Internet users, running a blog or a site. In addition, they have developed a certain habit of communicating about their disease and their daily life, enjoying making and reading testimonials. A correlation therefore appears between expert patients and the use of digital tools. The objective of these interviews was also to evaluate the position of these expert patients to healthcare professionals: do they place themselves in opposition, in complementarity or in parallel with healthcare personnel, in short, how do they define their role as expert patients?

The aim of this chapter is therefore to understand the emergence of this new figure (the expert patient) in relation to contemporary changes in the professional healthcare sector, as well as to take stock of the discourse of promotion in relation to the reality of the practice of the expert patient. If the professionalization of the patient has been a given (section 6.2) over the last 30 years, its institutionalization has its origins in a complex intertwining of mutations, particularly societal and technological (section 6.3). Finally, beyond discourse and hopes, it will be important to understand how expert patients live out their role and practice their "profession", in complementarity with medical staff and relying heavily on a mastery of digital tools.

6.2. Mutating health care: the professionalization of the patient

A vast movement of changes has affected the sector since the 1980s, described as "health democracy". The patient is called upon to become, if not the equal of the doctor, at least in a situation of rebalancing: involved in his or her care, involved in care and decisions and benefiting from total transparency in his or her care with the availability of all information. The expert patient then appears to be both the consequence and the figurehead of this movement, to such an extent that she or he is now fully integrated into the healthcare institutions and has a diploma, thus attesting to skills and knowledge.

However, what can be described as the professionalization of the patient is the result of many factors that we need to come back to.

6.2.1. *General framework*

6.2.1.1. *Chronic diseases*

Chronic degenerative diseases were at the core of the health sector in the 20th century. The epidemiological transition, that is, the reduction in mortality owing to infectious diseases and the increase in mortality owing to so-called "chronic degenerative diseases", has had a profound impact on the medical sector. Since the 1960s, life expectancy has increased. People can now live for a long time with a disease that cannot be cured. This is all the more the case since this has also been the period during which medicine has begun to deal with many everyday problems (medicalization of everyday life). In this context, patients are considered incapable of governing themselves and are placed under the responsibility of the doctor. They are therefore patients who have been relieved of responsibility and made subject to medical authority [KLE 12]. The physician has full power and the patient her or his full trust, according to a paternalistic model.

In the 1980–1990s, with the exponential development of cancers and AIDS, the questioning of medicine and public health policies was at their peak. In addition, several political–medical affairs took place during the same period, accentuating the media coverage and criticism of health [MAR 10]. It is in this context that society must learn how to manage chronic diseases, diseases that cannot be treated (cancer, AIDS, Alzheimer's, etc.) and that cause inevitable physical and sometimes intellectual decline. The psychological, social and economic consequences are becoming significant in society: rising healthcare costs, ways of dealing with the end of life, changes in prevention through responsible behavior. Confidence in medical personnel and, more broadly, in science is shattered. This phenomenon is accentuated by the emergence of new forms of militancy and the development of ICT, which contribute to putting medicine under debate. From now on, the patient, individually or collectively, claims to be informed, and above all to be responsible for his or her care. The expert patients we met thus declared that they had encountered problems when they asked for information from healthcare personnel: "with personnel who were not available to exchange information and who did not understand my illness", problems linked "essentially to a lack of time". Some also reported being victims of "withholding information" and a "lack of information".

According to the World Health Organization (WHO), a "chronic disease" is a long-term condition that changes over time. Degenerative diseases are diseases in which one or more organs gradually degrade. A chronic degenerative disease is therefore a long-term, progressive disease in which one or more organs progressively degrade.

It is this type of pathology that is at the origin of the epidemiological transition. This term is used to describe changes over time in the causes of death: a decrease in mortality owing to infectious diseases and an increase in mortality owing to chronic degenerative diseases.

The Murray report published in December 2012 in the leading British medical journal *The Lancet* complemented the findings of the WHO. Transmissible, maternal, neonatal and nutritional diseases accounted for 25% of deaths in 2010 compared to 34% in 1990. At the same time, deaths from non-communicable diseases had increased from 57% to 65%. This reflects a change in the impact of major risk factors. Between 1990 and 2010, the number of deaths related to hunger decreased from nearly 1 million to 700,000 and those related to a lack of access to drinking water and poor hygiene conditions from over 700,000 to 340,000. At the same time, the number of deaths from diabetes almost doubled from 665,000 to 1.28 million and those related to metabolic risk factors (diet and physical inactivity) increased from 13.4 million to more than 18 million.

Box 6.1. *A perspective on chronic degenerative diseases*

6.2.1.2. *The patient at the center*

The healthcare system then becomes more patient-centered than disease-centered, leading to the end of a form of medical paternalism in favor of a patient/healthcare professional partnership. The term "contemporary patients" [FAI 06, KLE 12] refers to a set of scientific, technological and societal changes that have placed the patient at the center of the healthcare system. The willingness of patients to participate in the healthcare field is a reality, but there are ambiguities and contradictions.

EXPERT PATIENT.–

The expert patient is someone who, suffering from a chronic disease, has, over time, developed a detailed knowledge of his or her illness and has learned to live with it. The expert patient is above all an actor in her or his own health. Recently, they have been granted a status thanks to the implementation of university training (and degrees).

The expert patient gets involved with other people with the same chronic pathology as him or her. True experts in their pathologies, they have acquired a knowledge of medical language and expertise in the pathology that gives them legitimacy and credibility in the message they deliver.

Expert patients intervene as a complement and in collaboration with the healthcare team.

Not all patients become experts and not all contemporary patients become educators. Certain skills are necessary, hence the development of training courses. They have existed for a long time in the English-speaking world (such as the Expert Patient Program[1] in Great Britain, which has existed since 2001). They are increasing and becoming organized in France (e.g. Patient University at Sorbonne University). The Quebec model is undoubtedly the most successful in promoting patient expertise by proposing a partnership relationship between caregivers and expert patients [POM 15]. All these approaches aim to ensure that the scientific knowledge of professionals and the experiential knowledge of expert patients are taken into account in the act of care. However, the expert patients we met had difficulty in giving a precise definition of their role, while emphasizing its importance: "my role as an expert patient is very important within the clinic", says one of our expert patients. Others are more precise about their role: "I am a mediator between doctors and patients. I allow patients to better understand and interact with their doctor" or "I see myself as a facilitator. My role allows caregivers to have a better understanding of patients' lives. I also help patients to adopt a more autonomous posture."

This desire for patient investment goes beyond care and can have an impact on the organization of services and the governance of institutions. This is the challenge of health democracy: democratizing the health professional sector for the benefit of the patient; placing the patient at the heart of the system; allowing him or her – alone or represented by a group – not only to have a right of oversight, but also to act directly. In particular, patients are seen as relevant to improving care pathways. In Quebec, this is the objective of the *Direction collaboration et partenariat patient* (Guidance on patient partnership and collaboration) within the Partners in Care and Services program. This program makes professionals aware of patient intervention and patients receive training. While some patients are willing to put their skills at the service of the community on a voluntary basis, others are paid, furthering the idea of professionalizing the patient. In addition to remuneration, this professionalization makes it possible to give the expert patient an official status authorizing him or her to intervene in equal parts and as a complement to the care teams. In France, it was the 2002 law that allowed users to sit on supervisory boards or users' committees. At

1 Multi-week course sessions led by a chronically ill patient for his or her peers with the goal of helping patients self-manage their disease.

the departmental, regional and national levels, they are also present in regional health agencies and national health insurance funds.

The "rhetoric of the patient at the center" [BAS 10] has thus been present for several decades and refers to the different conceptions of the patient: sick person, patient, user, client, even consumer.

6.2.2. *The slow evolution of the patient's status and role*

The evolution from patient to expert patient was not direct. The term "patient" comes from the Latin *patiens*, meaning "to bear, to endure, to suffer". So etymologically, the patient is defined as passive in the face of the disease he or she is suffering from and in the face of the caregivers. The term "expert patient" reverses the situation by replacing the passive patient with an active patient.

6.2.2.1. *From invalid to patient*

Until the 19th century, medicine was certainly taught, but physicians were in competition with other "therapists": barbers, healers, herbalists, pharmacies and priests [FAU 93, GUI 09]. This was the era of patient-oriented medicine, at the sick person's bedside, at home. During the 19th century, experimental medicine appeared: theory and practice were combined in the knowledge of anatomy. It was still practiced at the sick person's bedside, but the sick person was now hospitalized. Medicine focuses on the disease (symptoms, clinical signs, care protocol) and no longer on the patient.

Throughout the 20th century, medicine was modernized. The patient's body was objectified and became a medium for diagnosis. The term "patient" replaced "invalid". Etymologically, "patient" in English means "person undergoing medical treatment".

As a result, if the passage from invalid to patient symbolizes the centrality of the patient, it is also the birth of care by the medical institution. This comes back to highlighting the establishment of networks of healthcare institutions, and the institutionalization of healthcare professionals, that is, to thinking of and implementing the entire organization of healthcare as a professional field and an economic sector. In doing so, a paternalistic model is established both from the point of view of healthcare management and from the point of view of economic organization, a model in which the patient is relieved of responsibility and is dependent on the doctor.

6.2.2.2. *The emergence of the contemporary patient*

After World War II, this paternalistic model was questioned by several elements. First, health was no longer reduced to medical logic alone. It aimed at more than just not being sick, but at a state of physical, mental and social well-being. The patient was seen as a person and his or her entire well-being needed to be taken into account. The hygienist approach was thus supplanted by an approach centered on the individual. The transmission of information now went through public health promotion authorities. These were the beginnings of public prevention policies and therapeutic education. These new elements required the intervention and training of new professionals. The cohabitation of healthcare personnel with these new personnel dedicated to health eventually led to the decompartmentalization of medical sciences in the 1970s. A vast network of people managing health programs was set up. Peer education was developed.

Continuing this trend, the 2000s were marked by the liberalization of medical information, characterized by an increase in the volume, circulation and speed of health information (see section 6.3). As a result, medical staff, health personnel and, especially, patients are very well informed. This is the contemporary patient. They are evolving in a context where they are now suffering from a chronic disease, and are therefore permanently ill, in a society that no longer wishes to grant a monopoly on care to biomedical players alone. At the end of the 20th century, all the elements were in place for the implementation of the first self-management initiatives. As a result, professionals taught patients techniques to promote their empowerment and reduce their dependence on the biomedical institution. On the basis of these principles, so-called "expert patient" programs are created. This concept quickly became an institutional fad. It reflects the desire to overturn expertise, which is no longer reserved for professionals. This new place of the patient was enshrined in law: in 1979, in European law with the European Charter for the Patient as Hospital User; and in France with the 2002 law on patients' rights and the quality of the healthcare system, centered on the notion of the user and health democracy. The notion of the user replaces that of the patient. It refers "to a conception of public service that gives rights and duties, and better still responsibilities, to those who benefit from services organized by the community" [LAS 07, p. 131].

With the professionalization of the patient status, a state (being sick) becomes a job. This evolution accompanies or illustrates the changes in the caregiver–patient relationship. It is the recognition that people who have learned to live with an illness have developed knowledge and skills that can be shared: "I know more about my illness than some caregivers and I am more able to talk about it than they are."[2] This trend is very much linked to the availability of an unprecedented amount of

---

2 Expert patient 1.

information. All the expert patients we met (100%) said they had looked for, are still looking for and disseminate information on one or more digital dispositives. They all declared they use the Internet several times a day. The tools used included search engines, specialized sites, discussion forums, blogs and social networks. Some 58% of them owned their own digital devices. It should be noted that this digital practice and the use of one's own digital device are, in all cases, prerequisites for training and for acquiring the status of expert patient. The latter is therefore indeed a digital expert patient.

Paradoxically, this patient who claims to be informed, which is in fact the case thanks to the development of online information, is also a patient who exchanges little information with healthcare staff: 57% of the expert patients we met said that they do not discuss health information found on different media with the healthcare staff. These results for 2019–2020 corroborate those of two surveys conducted among Internet users visiting the site Doctissimo. Whether in 2005 (first survey), in 2010 (second survey) or in 2019, patients are still hesitant to share the results of their search for information with healthcare personnel [ROM 07, ROM 12].

6.2.3. *The evolution towards health information*

The changes in health information are numerous[3]. First, the very nature of information has evolved from *medical* to *health information*. Then, the increased accessibility to this information has made it totally overwhelming. Finally, health, like all other fields, has been won over by a social practice that has developed with the digital age: swapping life stories. Patients can now exchange information with other patients or different healthcare personnel, or even multiple activist groups through blogs, forums, sites and social networks. Dialog is therefore almost permanent, as is the production of information: important collectives are thus formed.

> LIFE NARRATIVES AND HEALTH.–
>
> A life narrative or storytelling consists of telling one's story, telling the story of one's life or a fragment of one's life. In the area of health, it is a matter of describing daily life with the illness, the treatment, the caregivers, the friends and family and so on.
>
> This kind of narrative, which has long existed in literature, has developed exponentially in the field of health, first with reality TV shows (1990s), and then with digital dispositives, such as blogs, sites or discussion forums (since the 2000s). This type of expression is halfway between testimonial and biography.

3 For more details, see [ROM 07, ROM 08, ROM 09, ROM 15].

The characteristic of health-related life narratives is that they allow their authors to free themselves by talking about themselves, and also to benefit their readers by allowing them to see that others are in the same situation and are experiencing the same thing.

The practice of life narratives or storytelling thus develops a link with the processes of resilience. Published on digital dispositives, they engage in interactivity and engender the creation of communities.

6.2.3.1. *Medical/health information*

It is now commonplace to use the Internet for health information. The first sites appeared in the mid-1990s and since then, their number has continued to grow. Health information is no longer controlled by doctors alone. The singular colloquium no longer pits a single professional holding the information against a supposedly ignorant patient.

In addition to the considerable growth in consumer health information, public health information is also growing. The public information project is part of a strategy to open up the administration to citizens in order to bridge the widening gap between citizens and their administration. ICT is invested with collaborative power and a mission of knowledge sharing [BEN 01, BON 03, CAR 01]. The development of the use of ICT is a key element of communication with and by professionals, and with and by patients, is being established on a permanent basis.

Beyond accessibility, it is the production of this information that has been liberalized and generalized, thereby multiplying the status of information producers. This category of information, traditionally scientific (produced, disseminated and controlled by the professional body of scientists) and public (produced and disseminated by the State), has become available to the general public. As public information, it was fully in line with the operating methods of public policies; as scientific information, it had to meet the precise criteria for evaluation and dissemination by the scientific community before being addressed to the general public. This is no longer the case: the production of health information is no longer the prerogative of either the medical sector or the public sector (the State). Medical information has, without doubt, been transformed into health information.

6.2.3.2. *A plethora of information*

This evolution accompanies the successive broadening of the very definition of health, notably by the World Health Organization. As a result, it is increasingly less about biomedical subjects and more about well-being issues, such as nutrition, or the evocation of living healthily instead of clinical elements. Health is becoming more social. Information is less medical and more health-related, less scientific and intended more for the general public, and it has left the specialized pages to become accessible to all media content. It has thus become more societal and more cross-cutting [ROM 08], and is also coveted by the content industries as it has large audiences [ROM 08, ROM 12]: health information for the general public is now totally overwhelming. This broadening of the conception of health towards well-being is a source of delight for publishers of press and audiovisual or multimedia content. There have never been so many press titles devoted to health, or so many specialized magazines or websites dealing with this topic. It is one of the very few print magazine sectors that remain economically profitable in France.

In the end, the patient is, at best, highly informed, as well as potentially over-informed or even misinformed, all the while claiming a less passive situation and seeking to get involved. The Internet users surveyed said that they consult these sites to "find people like them", "people who understand what I'm going through", "people who just talk"[4]. Expert patients described the information provided by healthcare workers as "too vague, inappropriate".

6.2.3.3. *A new form of information: life narratives*

In fact, most of the time, the consultation of health websites favors message boards, with Internet users declaring that they particularly appreciate testimonials, a non-professional word.

Although ancient, the development of so-called ordinary (i.e. lay) speech amplifies transformations. This movement must be seen in the context of a broader social movement, that of "forms of citizen involvement in the decisions that concern them […], one of the major features of the recent evolution of democratic regimes" [ROS 06, p. 301]. First, there was the question of "forms of organization and procedures designed to facilitate cooperation between specialists and laymen [and] to make visible and audible emerging groups without official spokespersons" [CAL 01, p. 60].

Subsequently, technical innovations have provided the opportunity for individual, unframed and interactive public expression: testimonials. The forms of self-expression are the success of Web 2.0, then Web 3.0. There are several explanations for this: first, the investment of content publishers and major media groups is linked to the profitable status of health [MAR 10]; second, this investment is favored by the absence of a binding legislative framework, unlike professional information; and third, this investment is favored by the trend towards individualization and the dematerialization of media. In addition, health, which

4 Interviews conducted with Doctissimo message board users in 2002, and then in 2007.

refers to a large extent to intimacy, is perfectly compatible with the practice of anonymity and the use of pseudonyms specific to a community Internet. Generating a consubstantial empathy, it provokes interactivity almost naturally. From then on, the sharing of experiences becomes widespread.

In Table 6.1, we summarize the results of two studies on the use of testimonials on television and the Internet [ROM 07, ROM 12]. Life narratives are changing the status of testimonials. From being illustrative in traditional media, they are becoming informative in Web 2.0 interactive dispositives. As a result, on the Doctissimo forum, testimonials account for about 50% of the exchanges, whereas the sharing of scientific information represents only 20%. The forum is a place where participants talk about their experience of the disease. Even if the Internet users declare themselves attached to a validation of scientific information, they also state that they do not want validation by "experts". In these community spaces, it is the individual's experience that is a guarantee if not of reliability, then at least of the interest and relevance of the information.

From then on, the patient becomes an expert in his or her pathology, as well as an expert in the art of talking about it and giving advice. At the border of the influential blogger, the expert patient emerges. This is the case of Beate Bartès and her website *Vivre sans thyroïde*[5] (Living without thyroid) or Estelle Lecointe, who has become the key contact for the medical community dealing with a rare and serious stomach cancer, gastrointestinal stromal tumor (GIST)[6]. Some 50.2% of the expert patients we surveyed believe they are influential, while 58% of them feel they benefit from an active community via their website or blog.

At the end of this section, we have explained the slow professionalization process of the patient, since the transition from invalid to patient, and then with the emergence of the expert patient. In the context of the epidemiological transition, a skill and knowledge are now recognized for patients living with their pathology long term. These contemporary patients rely on health information that is widely available on the Internet, but above all on a new form of expression: life narratives and the sharing of experiences between non-professionals. We asked expert patients about the use of life narratives: 58% of them said they use life stories, whether their own or those of others. This type of expression is "inevitable", "unavoidable on the Internet" or "the only way to really understand what the disease is". From this point of view, the expert patient can be analyzed as the result of several mutations and complex interactions.

5 www.forum-thyroïde.net.

6 http://ensemblecontrelegist.com.

A social field, whatever it may be, rarely changes by itself. Mutations are, in principle, the consequence of multiple interactions. Concerning the health field, irrespective of the will of patients to be at the heart of the system, whatever their desire for accountability, the acceptance of these claims stems from broader developments that we must now focus on.

	Illustrative testimonial	**Argumentative testimonial**	**Informative testimonial**
Appeared	19th century (popularization) to the present day	Mid-1980s to the present day	Late 1990s to the present day
Medium	Traditional press (scientific section, health section) Television and radio (health program)	Television and radio (company show or talk show) Traditional press (company section and policy section)	Internet (forum) Social networks Blogs
Aim	Dissemination Pedagogy	Proof Debate/accusation	Individual expression Life story
Tone	Didactic Technical and specialized	Compassionate Controversial	Emotive Solidarity Informative
Status	Example	Argument	Constitutes the message

Table 6.1. *Place and role of testimonials in health information*[7]

6.3. Societal changes and the emergence of the expert patient in the digital context

Since the post-World War II era, science has been widely questioned around the world. Medicine will also gradually be questioned. Forms of individualization of health practices and life choices such as the refusal of vaccination, the search for so-called alternative information on the Internet and the call for alternative medicine, among others, are also developing. These choices are expressed through new forms of activism.

7 Table designed by the author on the basis of several studies, already published in the journal *Communication* [ROM 12].

6.3.1. *New modalities of militancy*

6.3.1.1. *Challenging science and medicine*

Since the 1950s, positivism has come to an end and a critique of science and scientists has developed. Health is no exception to this movement. Medicine and its paternalistic model are questioned by medical institutions, patients, philosophers (Canguilhem) or social scientists, such as Goffmann or Foucault. The questioning takes different forms depending on the country and the period. At the beginning of the 20th century, the self-help movement emerged in the United States to break up with patient dependency. Its international echo contributed to the process of revaluing the patient and to the implementation of mechanisms to guarantee respect for people, benevolence, justice, equity and autonomy, first applied to research and then to the clinic.

In the 1990s, a new crisis of mistrust towards medicine as a result of media affairs reinforced skepticism. Patients became aware of the fallibility of health professionals, and physicians felt a devaluation of their status and a loss of legitimacy.

The new modalities of AIDS activism in the 1980s and 1990s also contributed to changing the role of the patient. Movements, inspired by civil rights struggles, did not hesitate to confront public authorities and enter into civil disobedience or take illegal actions.

In the end, this vast movement of questioning with heterogeneous modalities leads to a distrust of science and public authorities, a distancing from the physician's point of view, an affirmation of patients' identity and an affirmation of the role of associations.

6.3.1.2. *The role of associations*

The associations, which until then had accommodated paternalistic medicine, are now led by committed patients who assert their role and their knowledge. They intend to decide on the nature of their care [CAR 04]. The patient becomes a "social reformer" [BAT 09] and the concept of lay experts [EPS 95] is introduced with the idea of the need to recognize it. Madeleine Akhrich *et al.* proposed the notion of "patient knowledge" to qualify the knowledge of patients about their personal experience of a disease and their medical knowledge of this pathology [AKR 09]. Associations will play a central role in the deployment of patient knowledge by producing information [AKR 09, p. 75]. Mary Charoud [CHA 12] extends the notion of patient knowledge by emphasizing the collective and constructed nature of this knowledge. The patient knowledge of associations thus enables the design of specialized communication supports on different themes. During her doctoral work, she updated the different modes of action of these associations: first, action in terms of daily assistance to patients and families (which brings us back to the status of a recognized caregiver today); important work in the production and dissemination of information on diseases and their treatment; and finally, more "political" actions, to extend the action of the State (particularly on prevention), or to defend the rights of patients.

This work by associations, new forms of militancy and the questioning of scientific experts have led to the "slow emergence of a 'patient power'" that is gradually being institutionalized [HAS 99]. As a result, 85% of the expert patients we met are members of an association, sometimes with a leadership role. On average, they have been members of this association for 6.8 years, whereas they have been expert patients for an average of 1.6 years.

6.3.1.3. *The legal status of the patient*

The legitimacy of the patient has been legally shaped through regulatory and legislative texts of various forms (codes, charters, circulars, orders, directives, ordinances, laws, etc.). Patients' rights have developed in parallel with individual rights aimed at protecting patients against medical malpractice, as well as the right to social security, the humanization of hospitals, the rights of hospitalized patients and the right to information and consent of sick people. Patients' rights are thus not only recognized, but also extended.

Moreover, in the legal status of the patient there are multiple figures (individual, citizen, user, client, sick person, minor, family circle, disabled person, etc.) and a patient is considered to be in different situations (hospitalized, chronically ill, participant in research, on a one–off visit, etc.). This new patient and his or her rights thus adapt to the broadening of the definition of health.

It is within this framework that the political project of general legislation on the rights of the sick was developed in France in the 1980s and 1990s, and led in 2002 to the promulgation of a law on the rights of the sick and the quality of health systems, which has been constantly supplemented since then. The notion of *health democracy* was then introduced, structured around individual rights that concern the personal situations of patients and users, on the one hand, and collective rights that cover the collective, political, social and economic dimensions of the functioning of the health system and user participation, on the other hand [LAU 16].

If it responds to the wishes of the proponents of health democracy, this fundamental movement in favor of patients' rights is also an embodiment of democratic individualism, and of the transition to a very individual conception of health.

6.3.2. *Technological change and empowerment*

Blamed for the technicality of their vocabulary, the segmentation of care, the increasing focus on cost aspects and the lack of time given to patients, medicine and doctors are increasingly presented as dehumanized, with, in particular, a deterioration in the relationship between patient and doctor. An expert patient tells us about the importance of patient interaction: "[…] that the patient experience is irreplaceable. […] we are in the same emotional, psychological and expressive register. That our knowledge of the disease is embodied."[8] Another tells us that he was confronted with a "lack of information due to the fact that the caregiver presupposes that I am not able to understand certain technical terms, or that I don't need to."[9] In this case, and in a context where "patient power" tends to unite behind the notion of empowerment, the idea of the expert patient can be analyzed as an attempt to solve this crisis.

The patient is integrated into social networks, exchanges and learns about the disease. The power that the singular colloquium gave to the doctor is thus called into question. The principle of the singular colloquium (the "meeting of trust and conscience" according to the formula often attributed to Hippocrates), on which medical practice has been based since Antiquity, by making the physician the heart of the health system, is faltering under the effect of several setbacks: the reinforcement of patients' rights, developments in information and communication technologies, and societal transformations.

6.3.2.1. *Agency theory and asymmetry situation*

The patient–physician relationship has sometimes been analyzed using the agency theory (Ross; Jensen and Meckling): the doctor–patient relationship would be a situation where one individual depends on the action of another individual. The relationship would be unequal owing to an asymmetry of information in favor of the doctor and would lead to phenomena of adverse selection and moral risk (absent or incomplete information, difficulty in assessing the relevance of the doctor's decisions). The patient would thus defer to the doctor, leading to a paternalistic relationship where the patient is given little information by the doctor.

This view may be considered abusive in the sense that a number of safeguards (professional bodies such as a national council, peer review) must ensure that this does not happen. Moreover, if we can speak of an asymmetry of knowledge, it is difficult to support an asymmetry of information as ICT has made it possible to make a lot of information available, which reduces the effects of moral risk. Faced with a doctor, the patient's alternative is therefore to delegate the decision completely to

8 Expert patient 5, September 2, 2019.

9 Expert patient 3, August 26, 2019.

the doctor or to reduce the asymmetry of knowledge from which he or she suffers in order to "check" or at least try to appreciate the doctor's decisions. The expert patients we met stated that they look for information on the Internet because the "information is more precise and updated more frequently."[10] Patient empowerment in relation to the doctor can be individual or collective; it can take place in the interaction with the doctor or, on the contrary, in a totally parallel way, as the patient considers the information provided by the doctor too succinct or of insufficient quality.

In terms of information, legislation (Kouchner law of 2002, law of July 21, 2009) and the development of ICT have corrected the imperfect transmission of information by the doctor. The Internet not only provides people with information and opinions that may be contrary to national health policy, but it also allows them to share their opinions with others and build alliances to challenge these same policies. The role of the Internet is all the more important since several studies have shown, for example, that patients are re-examining their medical prescriptions based on the information or experiences they consult [BIS 01]. This type of action does not necessarily correspond to a discrediting of the physician, but rather to the patient's willingness to make a personal commitment, to take responsibility for his or her care.

It remains to be seen whether the reduction in information asymmetry has corresponded to a reduction in knowledge asymmetry. Non-specialists in information communication tend to think so. Giddens, in 1991, argued that e-health, by modifying patients' health knowledge, could lead to a democratization of lay/professional relationships. Specialists in information communication sciences, especially those who have worked on reception and appropriation, obviously do not take this step. There is certainly a better dissemination of information, but the improvement in knowledge remains uneven owing to differences in appropriation and differences in the assimilation capacity of the general public. Here, we are touching on one of the major confusions with digital technology: that the provision of information would mechanically increase knowledge. However, these are two very different processes and there is no automatic link between the two.

The information deficit has been considerably reduced thanks to the deployment of online health information. The knowledge deficit remains random depending on individuals and their ability to transform information into knowledge. Nevertheless, the availability of information has generated discussions on the role of the Internet in the patient–physician relationship. "On the one hand, there are those who believe that the Web contributes to the accountability of patients and their emancipation from the exclusive authority of the medical profession; on the other hand, there are those who fear the impact on the patient of a breach of the contract of trust, the poor

10 Expert patient 3.

quality of information, the power of charlatans or 'interested parties'" [MEA 10, p. 41]. Moreover, the patient's participation in the sphere of knowledge (participation rather than control) and the decision-making process brings multiple actors into the game. In the past, knowledge was only available to physicians and institutional sites. Today, individual patient sites, blogs, forums, association sites, etc. are all involved. There are therefore a multitude of channels for transmitting information and/or knowledge.

6.3.2.2. *Peer support and empowerment*

The production of information by non-professional actors is at the heart of change. As a result, during the 1980s, with the AIDS epidemic, patients came together to create associations. They became militant and combined the production of information, the denunciation of public policies, publications, therapeutic trials and more. Some are so knowledgeable that they become experts who are consulted by researchers and influence public health policy. From there, the status of the peer helper is developing around the world: as early as the 1990s in the United States, in 2005 in Quebec, and in 2012 in France with the World Health Organization collaborating centers for the implementation of peer helper health mediators. The concepts of recovery, empowerment and peer support have been around for a long time. It is only recently that healthcare professionals have begun to take an interest in them. Patient expertise is referred to as experiential knowledge, as well as intimate knowledge.

The framework of a peer-to-peer relationship is based on the identification of one person, the recipient, with another person, the peer-helper, on the basis of common experiences.

Today, more and more users of the healthcare system are advocating a reappropriation of their power and a willingness to extricate themselves from a logic of dependency, disability and chronicity. They call for the principle of self-determination (empowerment) and the recognition of mutual aid between peers. In our so-called "risk society" (Ulrich Beck), we are all engaged in a search for information on potential risks that could transform or affect our lives. The participation of citizens in decision-making has two distinct axes. One concerns the involvement of citizens in what directly affects the management of their own health problems (or those of their loved ones). The other concerns, more generally, citizen involvement in decisions relating to the health system itself and its organization. Peer support and the expert patient fall within the first axis only.

Being a "health" actor is something else entirely. As a citizen who votes, pays taxes and health insurance, you have a say in the major orientations of your country's healthcare system. This is what the proponents of health democracy are calling for, but its actual implementation is encountering a great deal of resistance and is still not up to date.

The emergence of expert patients is therefore part of a vast movement to democratize science [COU 97], itself linked to the loss of confidence in the power of science and in the ability of experts to save lives. At the same time, public health policies are trying to promote the idea that citizens must be informed of risks in order to make decisions about their diet, exercise and so on [COU 97]. At the same time, public health policies are trying to promote the idea that citizens need to be informed of risks in order to make decisions about their diet, exercise and so on in an effort to empower individual citizens.

6.3.3. *Therapeutic patient education: the unthought-of digital culture and literacy*

Emerging in the 1930s first for diabetes, therapeutic patient education (TPE) brings together intervention practices in the care relationship, support techniques and new care organization practices. They all aim to make patients more responsible. The expert patient is a direct result of the development of TPE.

The discourse on TPE knowledge and skills has been so pervasive since the 1990s that it is embodied in public actions (plans, laws, recommendations, etc.). However, although political science work emphasizes the strategies of actors in the relationship to the "referential" [MUL 06] by placing ideas at the center of the analysis, these ideas do not spread naturally. In the case of TPE, this knowledge has been developed by associations that have legitimized a new discipline and a new profession to the point of imposing them. It is therefore possible to read the emergence of expert patients in the light of a strategy for empowering professionals in therapeutic education. In doing so, it challenges the idea that the emergence of a more participatory patient is a sign of patient empowerment in relation to the medical field. In reality, the expert patient also comes from TPE, which itself finds its source within the health professionals themselves. From this point of view, the expert patient is the sign of a rupture within the health professionals between the supporters of paternalistic medicine and the supporters of change towards the patient.

The French Association for the Development of Therapeutic Education (*Association française pour le développement de l'éducation thérapeutique*, Afdet) plays a key role in the implementation of TPE and the emergence of expert patients. It produces and disseminates theoretical and practical knowledge in the field of French therapeutic education.

Three WHO collaborating centers for patient education exist in Europe, in Leuven, Geneva and Paris 13. These three centers have marked the institutional structuring of the TPE field. In France, the work of the Paris 13 research team in educational sciences has informed French policies in this field. Educational sciences have played a major role in the development of TPE, leading Nicolas Guiramand in 2015 to speak of a "pedagogization of care".

In 1998, national impetus was given to the development of patient education by the new Director General of Health, cardiologist Joël Ménard, who made it one of his priority objectives. In 1999, the accreditation manual for healthcare institutions published by the French health authority, *Agence nationale d'accréditation et d'évaluation*, included health education, while patient education was included in the circular message on diabetes management. From 2000 onwards, these initiatives foreshadowed the emergence of a political will, which was reflected in the announcement of several public policies advocating the development of patient education.

In 2007, a first methodological guide for therapeutic education was published by the French Health Authority, *Haute autorité de santé,* and the French National Institute for Education and Health, *Institut national pour l'éducation et la santé,* in order to streamline increasingly successful practices and training. Afdet's promotion of patient education in diabetology is becoming a demand for institutional therapeutic education, extended to all chronic diseases. A paradox should be noted: while expert patients have all developed daily digital practices, while most of them have developed digital tools that they claim to use to create a community of dialog and work on resilience, no digital training is provided as part of therapeutic education. The digital is the big missing element in therapeutic education training.

As the law makes training for healthcare workers involved in therapeutic education programs mandatory, demand for training from Afdet is increasing significantly. This association has thus had a lasting impact on TPE in France by imposing its vision (and its training) of therapeutic education and promoting the emergence of expert patients. The expert patient is therefore also the result of this struggle.

After the rise of TPE, a new concept emerged: the expert patient. Drawing on his or her experience of living with the disease on a daily basis, he or she represents a vital resource, both for medical teams and for other patients. Therapeutic education programs are flourishing in the management of many chronic diseases (diabetes, cardiovascular disease, respiratory failure, kidney failure, etc.). The involvement of patients in therapeutic education programs, followed by actions for other patients, has aroused the interest of the public health authorities. The latter then decided to include them in their advisory and decision-making bodies, to involve patients in

health decisions concerning their disease. As of 2009, they became mandatory in the management of all chronic diseases and are a priority for national public health policies.

In France, the notion of the expert patient is only beginning to emerge. In hospitals, it is gradually taking over from therapeutic education programs. However, these patients must receive specific training to become expert patients and transmit their knowledge to other **patients** and healthcare teams.

Faced with this need for training, the Patients' University, created in 2009 within the Pierre and Marie Curie University (now Sorbonne University), is the first **pedagogical system** in France that integrates expert patients into university courses on therapeutic education.

6.4. Conclusion

To conclude, we can affirm that the figure of the expert patient has historically been built up bit by bit. This is the result of the concordance of complex mutations: a society in a crisis of confidence with regard to its scientists and doctors; a context of chronic illness that sees people ill for longer; the explosion of ICT that has led to a situation of everyone, let alone the patient, being over-informed; the questioning of the singular colloquium opposing a knowledgeable doctor and a passive and obedient patient; internal struggles within doctors, some of them wishing to break with the paternalistic model; the importance of the patient's role as an expert in the field of medicine; the need to be able to understand the patient's needs and to be able to make informed decisions; therapeutic education and the pedagogization of care; and finally, new forms of activism that have claimed a central place for the patient in the healthcare system.

Our hypothesis is that the status of the expert patient has developed at the heart of important societal and technical changes. In this context, the promises of digital technology play a central role. It emerges from our study (which needs to be extended to be confirmed) that patients who become expert patients are integrated into the associative environment and connected for a long time, with a certain familiarity with storytelling. They have regular digital habits and are generally owners of a dispositive of digital expression, such as a website, blog or social network account. They first broadcast testimonials and storytelling, and then practice online consulting before training as expert patients. They readily declare that they feel influential and have developed a community. Even if this study should be extended to a larger cohort, it seems that the expert patient is someone who is digitally accustomed to life storytelling (habitual use but without training), empathy and advice.

It is also certain that the emergence of this figure of the expert patient goes hand in hand with the diffusion of democratic and neoliberal values in the health system. Autonomy, self-determination, the responsibility of the individual, his or her ability to exert an influence on matters that concern him or her (empowerment), to identify and satisfy his or her needs, to solve his or her problems and to control his or her life are emblematic values of contemporary individualism [GAG 14].

There is a disturbing concordance here with the changes in prevention policies aimed at breaking with the principle of collective care and the principle of collective solidarity in health care. Risk behaviors are now being singled out in terms of prevention, and the enactment of standards to determine what is risky and what is not. This is a trend that has been apparent in recent years in the changes in prevention, which is increasingly oriented towards the indictment of so-called risk behaviors and the emphasis on risk factors [ROM 13]. Will differentiated care soon be established? Indeed, if pathologies are attributable to individual behaviors, for the administration and for society, it will not be long before insurance companies produce differentiated treatments according to our behaviors. By moving from collective and solidarity-based care, the healthcare system would move towards individual care and responsibility (guilt-inducing?).

The reminder of these transformations should not obscure the fact that exclusive medical authority is far from having disappeared. Moreover, expert patients themselves do not at any time show any willingness to oppose or challenge this authority. They all declare that they are "in complementarity", "in parallel" or even "in partnership" with medical personnel.

6.5. References

[AKR 09] AKRICH M., MEADEL C., RABEHARISOA V., *Se mobiliser pour la santé, des associations de patients témoignent*, Presses de l'École des Mines, Paris, 2009.

[BAS 10] BASZANGER I, "Une autonomie incertaine : les malades et le système de soins", in HIRSCH E. (ed.), *Traité de bioéthique*, Érès, Toulouse, 2010.

[BAT 09] BATAILLE P., "La décennie des malades ?" *Les Tribunes de la santé*, vol. 25, no. 4, pp. 63–68, 2009.

[BEC 01] BECK U., *La société du risque ; sur la voie d'une autre modernité*, Aubier, Paris, 2001.

[BEN 01] BENGHOZI P.-J., "Technologies de l'information et organisation, de la tentation de la flexibilité à la centralisation", *Gestion*, vol. 2, no. 2, pp. 61–80, March–April 2001.

[BIS 01] BISSELL P., Ward, P.R., Noyce, P.R. "The dependent consumer: Reflections on accounts of the risks of non-prescription medicines", *Health*, vol. 5, no. 1, pp. 5–30, 2001.

[BON 03] BONNEVILLE L., La mise en place du virage ambulatoire informatisé comme solution à la crise de productivité du système socio sanitaire au Québec (1975–2000), Sociology PhD thesis, Université du Québec, Montreal, 2003.

[CAL 01] CALLON M., *Agir dans un monde incertain. Essai sur la démocratie technique*, Le Seuil, Paris, 2001.

[CAR 01] CARRÉ D., LACROIX J.-G., *La santé et les autoroutes de l'information. La greffe informatique*, L'Harmattan, Paris, 2001.

[CAR 02] CARRÉ D., Régulation sociale de la diffusion des TIC, HDR thesis, Université Stendhal-Grenoble 3, Grenoble, 2002.

[CAR 04] CARRIBURU D., MENORET M., *Sociologie de la santé, institutions, professions et maladies*, Armand Colin, Paris, 2004.

[CHA 12] CHAROUD M., Stratégies de communication et évolutions sociales : le cas des associations de patients, PhD thesis, Université de Grenoble Alpes, Grenoble, 2012.

[COU 97] COUCH S.R., KROLL-SMITH S., "Environmental movements and expert knowledge: Evidence for a new populism", *International Journal of Contemporary Sociology*, no. 34, pp. 185–210, 1997.

[EPS 95] EPSTEIN S., "The construction of lay expertise: AIDS activism and the forging of credibility in the reform of clinical trials", *Science, Technology and Human Values*, vol. 20, no. 4, pp. 408–437, 1995.

[FAI 06] FAINZANG S., *La relation médecins-malades : information et mensonge*, PUF, Paris, 2006.

[FAU 93] FAURE O., *Les Français et leur médecine au XIXème siècle*, Belin, Paris, 1993.

[GAG 14] GAGNON E., CLEMENT M., DESHAIES M.H., "Sujets de droits : l'interprétation des droits des malades", *Sciences sociales et santé*, vol. 32, no. 1, pp. 5–28, 2014.

[GID 91] GIDDENS A., *Modernity and Self-Identity*, Polity Press, Cambridge, 1991.

[GID 07] GIDDENS A., "Une nouvelle gamme de risques spécifiques de la modernité", *Problèmes politiques et sociaux*, no. 941, 2007.

[GRO 07] GROSJEAN S., BONNEVILLE L., "Logiques d'implantation des TIC dans le secteur de la santé", *Revue française de gestion*, no. 172, pp. 145–15, 2007.

[GUI 09] GUILLEMAIN H., "Devenir médecin au XIXème siècle", *Annales de Bretagne et des Pays de l'Ouest*, vol. 116, no. 3, pp. 109–123, Available at: http://abpo.revues.org/501 [Accessed 02/07/2019], 2019.

[HAB 62] HABERMAS J., *L'espace public. Archéologie de la publicité comme dimension constitutive de la société bourgeoise*, Payot, Paris, 1962.

[HAS 99] HASENTEUFEL P., "Vers le déclin du "pouvoir médical" ? Un éclairage européen : France, Allemagne, Pays-Bas", *Pouvoirs*, no. 89, 1999.

[KLE 12] KLEIN A., "Contribution à l'histoire du "patient" contemporain, l'autonomie en santé : du self-care au biohacking", *Histoire, médecine et santé*, no. 1, pp. 115–128, 2012.

[LAS 07] LASCOUMES P., "L'usager dans le système de santé : réformateur social ou fiction utile ?" *Politiques et management public*, vol. 25, no. 2, pp. 129–144, 2007.

[LAU 16] LAUDE A., TABUTEAU D., *Les droits des malades*, PUF, Paris, 2016.

[LOA 99] LOADER B.D., "Informational health networks: Health care organisations in the information age", in PURDY M., BANKS D. (eds), *Health and Exclusion; Collaborators and Victims in Health Care*, Routledge, London, 1999.

[MAR 10] MARCHETTI D., *Quand la santé devient médiatique. Les logiques de production de l'information dans la presse*, Presses Universitaires de Grenoble, Grenoble, 2010.

[MEA 10] MEADEL C., AKRICH M., "Internet tiers nébuleux de la relation patient-médecin", *Les Tribunes de la santé*, vol. 4, no. 29, pp. 41–48, 2010.

[MUL 06] MULLER P., "Quand les politiques publiques dévoilent les rapports de domination", *Politique européenne*, vol. 3, no. 20, pp. 141–145, 2006.

[OLI 06] OLIVESI S., *Sciences de l'information et de la communication, objets, savoirs, discipline*, Presses Universitaires de Grenoble, Grenoble, 2006.

[PIE 07] PIERRON J.-P., "Une nouvelle figure du patient ? Les transformations contemporaines de la relation de soins", *Sciences sociales et santé*, vol. 25, pp. 43–66, 2007.

[POM 15] POMEY M.-P., "Le Montreal model : enjeux du partenariat relationnel entre patients et professionnels de la santé", *Santé Publique*, hors-série, pp. 41–50, 2015.

[ROM 07] ROMEYER H., "La santé à la télévision : émergence d'une question sociale", *Question de communication*, no. 11, pp. 51–70, 2007.

[ROM 08] ROMEYER H., "Tics et santé : entre information médicale et information de santé", *Tic&société*, vol. 2, no. 1, Available at: www.ticetsociete.org, 2008.

[ROM 11] ROMEYER H., Pour une approche communicationnelle du processus de publicisation : le cas des questions de santé, HDR, Université Grenoble Alpes, Grenoble, 2011.

[ROM 12] ROMEYER H., "La santé en ligne : au-delà des enjeux d'information", *Communication*, vol. 30, no. 1, 2012.

[ROM 13] ROMEYER H., "Pour une approche interdisciplinaire de la prévention", *Communication & Langages*, no. 176, pp. 33–47, 2013.

[ROM 15] ROMEYER H., "Médiatisation et publicisation des sujets de santé", in BURGER M., MERMINOD G. (eds), *L'expertise dans les discours de santé – Cahiers de l'ILSL*, no. 44, Université de Lausanne, Lausanne, 2015.

7

Towards an Info-communication Categorization of Expertise in Online Health Communities

7.1. Introduction

Our post-industrial societies are defined, in particular, by a revolution in our relationship with knowledge, increased by the generalization of communications linked to the multiplication of ICT. Information from various sources is coming into opposition on different subjects, especially health. Defiance of State authority is becoming widespread as health scandals emerge: Chernobyl, the Mediator and, more recently, Lubrizol in Rouen. Official expertise no longer enjoys consensus and is in competition with others. These other forms of expertise win the approbation of a growing part of the public as mistrust of public institutions increases. The processes that lead to the legitimation of certain forms of expertise resonate with this mistrust. We support our proposal by studying the use, by a community, of forums dedicated to a socially acute question: the production and use of therapeutic cannabis. In this chapter, we propose a typology that makes it possible to return to what constitutes the nature of expertise, where it can be deployed and, above all, to which legitimation process(es) it is linked. We propose a schematization of these forms of expertise according to a profile that shows the processes of recognition and legitimation through which it passes.

The rest of this chapter will enable us to describe the crises that expertise is going through (section 7.2), particularly in the context of online health communities by questioning their relationship with the medical authorities (section 7.3). We will establish the need for an info-communicational definition, in tension between three

---

Chapter written by Stéphane DJAHANCHAHI, Olivier GALIBERT and Benoit CORDELIER.

modes of legitimation that seem to us to be decisive in qualifying the experts who express themselves in these spaces (section 7.4). Finally, we will propose a scheme for validating the expertise of the members of these online communities (section 7.5).

7.2. The crises of expertise in research in information and communication sciences

In our research, we approach experts as a form of reification of the legitimation of knowledge, because they make tangible, through their diagnoses, the application of legitimized knowledge. This application thereby legitimizes the knowledge that is at its origin. The experts thus possess theoretical knowledge and experience that they are able to use in a given situation to propose a diagnosis and a solution. This solution must win the approval of the other actors since the expert possesses and mobilizes the adequate knowledge. However, recent crises have shown us that the very way expertise is perceived is no guarantee of consensus: the questioning of the use of GMOs, vaccination and the human origin of climate change have brought with them their share of actors invited into the public debate as experts. This diversity of expert profiles has emerged in the media from a desire for impartiality on their part, particularly on socially acute questions, issues on which there is no scientific consensus, which are of interest to society as a whole and which bring different forms of knowledge into dialog, such as reference scientific knowledge, professional knowledge or social knowledge [SIM 08, p. 185].

LEGITIMACY AND EXPERTISE.–

The notion of expertise refers to an individual's ability to propose a diagnosis informed by legitimate knowledge in a given situation. According to Yves Trépos, depending on the situation, it can be used as a decision-making aid, but it can also have an incentive dimension [TRE 06, p. 17]. This incentive dimension can be compared to the institutional dimension of the expert in Robert Castel, who is then an actor who is no longer simply mandated for a diagnosis, but who is able to intervene to "incite" people to consider a problem in a certain way, according to a certain analytical framework different from the framework initially prescribed [CAS 85, p. 92]. For health issues, this is mainly distinguished between institutional expertise (whose credibility comes from the perceived image of the institution) and experiential expertise (whose credibility comes from the individual's experience). "Credibility is the result of the impression of validity and legitimacy given by the Internet user to the information he or she consults" [VIG 18, p. 149]. Legitimacy is a quality that underpins power and justifies the obedience that is owed to it[1]. This is an indispensable attribute of expertise that refers to the notion of authority. For Max Weber, the recognition of legitimacy has

1 https://www.universalis.fr/encyclopedie/legitimite/.

three origins: traditional, charismatic and rational-legal [WEB 13, p. 126]. These criteria are linked to the notions of experiential or institutional credibility and are dimensions to be taken into account when considering the legitimacy of an expert's status [VIG 18, pp. 149–150]. On the one hand, the recognition of an expertise will depend on the legitimacy of those who claim it in the eyes of those who receive it. On the other hand, the fact of using expertise testifies to its authority and helps to legitimize it. The quality of the diagnosis resulting from an expertise may therefore be independent of its legitimacy in the eyes of certain actors concerned by this same diagnosis.

7.2.1. *The question of expertise in the face of the diversity of forms of knowledge mobilized in socially relevant issues*

The nature of socially relevant issues means that they need to be addressed by actors at different levels in society, including scientists, as well as other actors. For example, discussions have pitted individuals with very different careers against each other. The term *career* here covers two notions. The first, traditional, meaning refers to the professional career of individuals, integrating their training and experience. The second, in the sense of Becker [BEC 85, p. 47], contains a dimension of learning from a practice, which is certainly established, but which can take place outside the typical and recognized frameworks of society. It is part of what he calls deviant practice, which can be informal, or even hidden from a part of society, shared by a restricted group of individuals. This second notion implies a development of expertise that is not only aimed at the efficiency of rational decision-making but also at the defense of particular or even community interests. Experts from the IPCC (Intergovernmental Panel on Climate Change) therefore had been able to stand up to lobbyists, doctors to presidents of parents' associations, agricultural researchers to representatives of farmers' unions, specialists in gambling addiction to gamblers, bloggers and so on. All of them proclaim their own expertise on the subject they are speaking about. Our purpose here is to highlight the fact that there is no single form of expertise that can bring consensus to the debate. Expertise does not only function as an aid to decision-making on a technical choice, but it also brings with it, in our information society, a set of representations and beliefs that are lent to the people who exercise it and on which they rely. Sintomer describes it thus [SIN 08, p. 125]:

> Expert opinion can no longer be taken at face value, because [experts] regularly make mistakes, because the solutions they propose will inevitably lead to unforeseen problems, but also, and more profoundly, because their expertise is influenced by cultural or political factors that are far from neutral.

Since the expert cannot position himself as the sole and absolute reference, researchers in the humanities have questioned the different characteristics that define the expert and have come to propose different qualifications and taxonomies [BOU 02, CAS 85, ETI 13, EPS 95, GRI 10, LAP 16, VIS 92]. As far as we are concerned, we will see in this chapter that the types of expertise, among others academic, technical-professional, experiential, lay, proximity and citizen, to propose a first, non-exhaustive list of those that can be of interest to socially relevant issues in the field of health, and that overlap and diverge on certain points.

It is difficult to provide an exhaustive list of definitions of expertise in the social sciences and humanities, as they differ across scientific disciplines and research objectives. As a result, if there is a dominant expertise, we could speak of *counter-expertise* [TRE 02, p. 12], but this would limit us to an oppositional approach to political games, whereas we postulate that it is the diversity of expertise that enriches the debate in the Habermasian perspective in which we are engaged. In this perspective, the existence of conditions that allow arguments to be debated, in a reasonable argumentation and in their diversity, is the basis of the conditions for the existence of the public sphere. Only the recognition of the possible diversity of forms of expertise is not acquired. A physician, for example, will find it difficult to recognize the expertise of patients, when they may come to be considered as "lay expert patients" [GRI 10, p. 91] or even "institutionalized or professionalized expert patients". As a result, as Salman and Topçu point out: "[lay expertise is a] notion that is neither stabilized nor neutral – including for the analyst – and which is the subject of debate among the actors it is intended to designate" [SAL 15, p. 164].

The issues of health information, particularly of lay origin, disseminated online have been addressed for questions of legitimacy and power [VIG 18, p. 157]. "The main issue of health information on the Internet is not so much the quality and rigor of the information, but rather the ability of the actors to attract the attention of Internet users." Beyond their visibility and influence, it is these conditions that allow individuals to be recognized as experts that interest us here. Spaces of exchange such as specialized forums, which we will consider restricted public spheres [MIE 10, p. 127], host processes that legitimize knowledge resulting from communicational processes that can lead certain individuals to a validation of their expert status by other actors in the observed space.

By recalling the issues and tensions related to the development and recognition of online expertise on health issues, we will highlight the challenges of an info-communicational understanding of it, particularly within online health communities. The methodology that allows us to support our argument comes from the PhD thesis work (in progress) of one of the authors. An interdisciplinary work, it is based on an ethnographic approach of different discussion forums where cannabis growers (people who cultivate cannabis for their own consumption or that of their relatives) meet, and on an analysis of sites that share informational resources on the same themes, as well as on semi-directive interviews with users of these forums and health professionals. This chapter is mainly based on the results of the ethnographic study.

7.2.2. *The place of expertise in info-communication and community-based online knowledge mediation dispositives*

The diversity of information sites, but especially the exchange platforms resulting from the so-called social or collaborative Web, which are used to share knowledge and experiences on health topics, leads ICS researchers to observe the forms and norms of socialization that result from them. It is therefore the epistemological conditions that we will use that will allow us to recognize the conditions for validating the production of expertise and thus the production of knowledge. These conditions of production invite us to link the e-health communities to various socio-technical means of sharing communications (such as forums, message boards, information, opinions, their links with politics, health institution, etc.), in the work of constructing this research object.

In the questioning of what differentiates an object of research from a concrete object [DAV 04, p. 31], expertise could appear at first sight to be a concrete object. It could easily be linked to our research object, by considering it to be a quality of certain members of online health communities. They would put their expertise forward in formulating one proposal or affirm it by criticizing another. However, expertise from different backgrounds regularly clash. The very definition of expertise has given rise to a wealth of academic activity on the subject (take, for example, the CRESAL round table in 1985 and the critical dictionary of expertise in 2015). This shows, apart from the fact that it has been of interest to social science researchers for decades, that its perception is not self-evident. Today, there seems to be a consensus that the traditional view of the expert – a specialist recognized by an institution as an authoritative means of solving a problem – is too restrictive to understand their role and the tensions that their existence creates in society.

In the field of health, the experience of patients from their lived experience of illness brings a personal and experiential dimension to the construction of expertise. Those qualified as "lay experts" have been able to appropriate specific knowledge, in mediation processes, between the information provided by doctors, their own experience and the information they may have at their disposal. The mediation of knowledge can be understood as "all the media and interactional processes that contribute to the construction, sharing, dissemination and even confrontation of socially institutionalized knowledge" [BON 16, p. 5]. The online collaborative spaces that are developing in the prevailing context of the digital society therefore multiply the number of spaces and channels that facilitate these media processes.

A new form of expertise is emerging and developing on the Internet, on certain forums dedicated, in particular, to the misuse of drugs, to cite one that has been studied specifically for these issues. Some participants appear to be "experts" because of their mastery of the terms and their knowledge of the effects and dosages, and thanks to their seniority [ORA 13, p. 88]. The forums in which our study takes place host groups that aim to develop their skills, as well as to share their experiences (of growing or processing cannabis). This sharing of experiences and their approval by the collective helps to legitimize the knowledge that has made it possible to develop or improve the technique used, according to theoretical and empirical criteria. These technical questions are then discussed by the rest of the collective, which we envisage within the framework of the virtual community theory that we will describe below.

MEDIATION OF KNOWLEDGE AND POPULARIZATION OF SCIENCE.–

Knowledge mediation refers to the action of sharing and making intelligible knowledge from at least two different origins. It can be similar to a form of diffusion and sharing of knowledge between individuals (experts or not) with different specialties. It includes, but is not limited to, the popularization of science. The latter refers to the act of conveying scientific information to the general public. It then designates, in particular, didactic processes that make specific knowledge, described in the technical language of experts and specialists, accessible to laypeople who do not master it. For health issues, mediation thus integrates horizontal exchanges (between laypeople or between specialists), as well as vertical processes that make specific knowledge accessible and that are carried out by specialists. Popularization, meanwhile, implies the status of different actors (laypeople and experts or specialists and the general public). Medical information (from professionals) and health information for the general public can be found on the Internet and social media [ROM 08, p. 30]. This general public information can be scientific information popularized by specialists, but it can also come from personal testimonials from outside any institutional framework. The dissemination of this information modifies the mediation process of health knowledge, which is adjusted by integrating the experience and testimony of the individual as a guarantee of credibility [ROM 08, p. 40].

7.3. Info-communicational theory of the online community link as a sociotechnical context for the deployment of online expertise

In order to analyze a health community, we first need to define it and understand what constitutes it. Our approach thus obliges us to categorize in it what we call an info-communication perspective, as we question the collective in the different mediations through which it is created, developed or transformed.

First, we choose to link it as an online community to the typical ideal of the virtual community [GAL 14]. This implies considering the members participate in an online community by submitting to the ethics of Habermasian discussion, in a logic of Maussian gift, in connection with a certain search for recognition as in the perspective of Axel Honneth. This ideal model must be considered, on the one hand, an emancipatory promise to user-members, and, on the other hand, the optimistic ideological form aimed at ideally normalizing interactions in digital collectives to make them more effective in the eyes of the info-communication objectives set by community management.

Researchers interested in social health networks have questioned the community dimension of certain online spaces where patients or caregivers meet: "The social network appears less a collective as such than a space where individuals who may share the same objectives come together" [ORO 11, p. 105]. In our case, we see a community dimension clearly displayed on the system and claimed by the members. The forum serves the community for sharing experiences, of course, but the durability of the exchanges over time and their convivial dimension remain essential. The following excerpt illustrates, using the metaphor of a ship and its crew, the community spirit that exists and is encouraged by the members. The welcome messages from the forums that we observe constitute a true "editorial line" representative of the alternative therapeutic orientation. They are also often mentioned when a member does not comply with the rules governing exchanges.

> Hello everyone and welcome aboard!
>
> If you're reading this, it's because you've decided to get on board and share our adventures; which you'll see are a compilation of nearly a decade of all kinds of buds and forms of cannabis deliriums as varied as they are exciting.
>
> Only to be part of such an old crew, there is a certain way to shape your presence and participation. We are all here because passion has driven us to be here, and I think it's important to help newcomers to better integrate into this state of mind that gives wind to our sails.
>
> Here more than anywhere else perhaps, there is a style to adopt that will allow you to take leaps and bounds in learning about self-production but also to perfect your knowledge, to discover new

horizons, to cross the path of old sea dogs that will save you from many salient reefs, not to mention your place within the crew itself.[2]

7.3.1. *The ICS approach to health communities*

Health communities are therefore a preferred field of study for ICS researchers in that they involve many research themes that are dear to them: the mediation of knowledge, controversies, knowledge building, support and so on, all supported by various sociotechnical devices, which, once again, need to be described and understood.

There are studies of forums that host online communities that address health issues outside of, in addition to, or in opposition to, the medical arena – including the use of diverted drugs and anorexia communities [THO 11, p. 113, TUB 16, p. 99]. These forums address issues related to symptoms, and opinions on health behaviors and controversial topics such as alternative therapies. On forums that host communities of practice or interest, however, information exchanges are more specific, such as weight-loss strategies for pro-Ana sites or dosage advice for forums focusing on recreational drug detours. These topics fall into specific fields where experience is essential, as there is no *a priori* manual in these areas. The search for information and information sharing are the two main drivers of the discussion in these spaces, and some stakeholders, through the quality of the information they develop and the recognition they receive from other members, take on the role of expert [ORA 13, p. 101]. They participate in the construction of knowledge in their respective fields. The expertise they seem to possess is relative to their practice and comes from their experience. It is a mixture of theoretical information and empirical experimentation that defines expertise in this sense.

As we have just seen, online expert knowledge development processes orchestrated on CSAI (community and service applications on the Internet) have been studied, but controversy has a special place. Once again, it is the health authority's information on marketed molecules that is used as a reference to discourage use of the drug, because the information, particularly on side effects, contained in the package leaflet helps to guide use. We will see in section 7.3.2 that online communities dedicated to the cultivation and consumption of cannabis for therapeutic (but also recreational) purposes offer an area of great interest, particularly in the relationship that their members have with the messages of the health authority and the healthcare system. This terrain is all the more interesting as the place of cannabis is changing its status in health policy, moving from being

2 Excerpt from a page pinned in the "presentations" section of the forum, published on November 20, 2009.

solely a public health problem to being a solution, especially in cases of therapeutic deadlock.

7.3.2. *Specificity of the terrain and the need for a new qualification of expertise*

Research on online health communities can be enriched by a particular field that allows us to observe the logic of knowledge mediation that bypasses the health system's argument of authority. These forums make it possible to observe logics of creation, claiming and assertion of expertise for which the relationship to the health authority is central without becoming decisive, because the members completely free themselves from the official word – which denies the therapeutic benefit of using the product.

Herein, we study different forums on which members discuss various topics related to cannabis[3]. These spaces are not only oriented towards pro-legalization activism, nor are they exclusively focused on the therapeutic uses of cannabis. They do, however, support discussions that address these aspects in a direct way, with a vision moving away from the health authority. The issues that are addressed are broad enough to integrate, on the one hand, the relations to science, to knowledge that is established and in the process of being institutionalized, and then take into account the political context of development and expression of different scientific advances and care. On the other hand, the experiential dimension is central, similar to patient communities, sharing with the latter a dimension of support and mutual community aid. We are therefore talking about online communities, the aim of which lies in a form of development of well-being and a vision of emancipation of a healthcare system that does not meet all the expectations of its users, in particular by limiting access to certain treatments and to information about them.

The recommendations of the French National Agency for the Safety of Medicines (*Agence nationale pour la sûreté du medicament*, ANSM) are, however, in the process of removing this limitation on access to information. Indeed, based on a review of the international literature, it now considers experimentation with therapeutic cannabis desirable for the following indications[4]:

– in pain that is resistant to treatments (drug or non-drug) that are available;

– in certain forms of severe and drug-resistant epilepsy;

3 *Les Forums cannabiques francophones*: https://www.cannaweb.info/fcf/index.php, and the Cannaweed Community forums: https://www.cannaweed.com/forums.

4 List of indications retained by the *Comité scientifique spécialisé temporaire* and approved by the ANSM on December 13, 2018.

– within the framework of supportive care in oncology;

– in palliative situations;

– in the painful spasticity of multiple sclerosis.

These indications have been discussed by the users of these forums almost since their creation in 2002, notably in support of foreign scientific literature on cannabis, whose more recent results have encouraged the conclusions of the ANSM. The relationship to scientific knowledge that has been established there, in opposition to the health authority in the case of France, is of definite interest for observing the processes of legitimation of knowledge within CSAI. We can observe, as we did in the excerpt from the presentation section of the cannabis grower forums, the emancipatory dimension of the interactions in these systems. By their very existence, they allow members to disseminate health information that by definition would fall within the law if it encouraged the use of cannabis[5], thus allowing users to access knowledge and, consequently, self-determination. We recall that medical speech was constrained by the legal framework as to the supposed effects of cannabis that would not be harmful. However, for health issues, it is the representatives of the health authority who remain experts. This is what makes the situation different in France: there is no authority that talks about cannabis in the terms expected by users. From 1970 to 2018, the discourse of the health authority denied the therapeutic virtues of cannabis, in a desire to be consistent with the legislation on narcotics and to encourage the development of other care techniques considered more effective. There is therefore a multitude of historical sources on traditional uses, old medical textbooks, oral habits and traditions, as well as more or less well-documented medical uses that served until very recently as reference sources for the communities we observe, although some States have experimented with, supervised or simply authorized its use for therapeutic purposes. This multitude of sources also allows the emergence of statements of fact whose source cannot be traced and that are not based on anything reliable when put forward, but which sometimes serve as a basis for certain proposals: for example, the idea that the grafting of a hop plant on to a cannabis plant produced psychoactive substances when no scientific demonstration has ever supported this. Orienting the user between these different pieces of information is also central to the policy of other cannabis grower forums, as the following excerpt illustrates:

5 "The provocation to the offense provided for in Article L. 3421-1 or to one of the offenses provided for in Articles 222-34 to 222-39 of the Criminal Code, even if this provocation has not been followed up, or the fact of presenting these offenses in a favorable light is punishable by five years imprisonment and a fine of 75,000 euros." (Article L3421-4 of the French Public Health Code)

Hello, and welcome to CannaWeed!

Cannabis growing is a rigorous passion, which requires time and hard work. It will require many hours of research and reading before you can get started. Otherwise, you will risk errors, delays and spending money on inadequate equipment.

We put at your disposal many guides with files on the different growing methods, a beginners' tutorial to approach the different aspects of indoor growing step-by-step, tutorials, do-it-yourself projects to help you carry out your installation yourself, a FAQ section for frequently asked questions, and, finally, a CannaWiki that centralizes information.

You can (must) also use the search function (99% of the questions you will want to ask have already been posted at some point in the forum).[6]

7.4. Info-communication approaches to health expertise

Dominique Pestre invites us to consider expertise in a less technocratic, perhaps more democratic [PES 07, p. 40] and therefore inclusive dimension when others attempt to separate the types of expertise. An initial review of the types of expertise described in the literature allows us to make a list of those that can be observed around socially acute questions in the health field and that therefore influence mediation and decision-making processes. We have classified them according to the mode of legitimation of their knowledge and their spaces of expression.

Of course, expertise in one category may not be recognized by others: experiential knowledge does not have the value of academic expertise in the eyes of specialists in different fields, even if some are able to recognize its value as a decision-making aid.

With this in mind, the expert must always renegotiate their position in relation to other experts. This means that the *career* (in Becker's sense) of the expert is central. However, the highlighting of the expert's career obeys different strategies according to the actors.

These different careers refer to different modes of legitimation of expertise. The result is a diversity of profiles that are nevertheless qualified as "experts" wherever they are expressed. It seems useful to understand what these forms of expertise have in common and where they differ in terms of modes of legitimation, recognition and the spaces in which they can be asserted.

---

6 Excerpt from the "presentation" section of the Cannaweed forums published on March 23, 2013.

Medical research on the therapeutic benefits of cannabis

The increase in research on the therapeutic applications of cannabis is echoed in the growing understanding of the role of cannabinoids in the body. Indeed, endogenous cannabinoids and their receptors constitute a physiological communication system regulating many aspects of the human body's functioning. These receptors have been identified from 1988 onwards following studies on the action of the main active ingredient of cannabis, THC, which was discovered as early as 1964 by Raphael Mechoulam, an Israeli chemist and professor of medicine. The study of the therapeutic applications of cannabis is today a very dynamic field of medical research, particularly in the fight against cancer, in terms of supportive care and also for the antitumor activity of certain cannabinoids such as THC and CBD [VEC 20, p. 24]. Cannabinoids also have analgesic, anti-emetic, anti-inflammatory and antipsychotic properties [GRO 03, p. 349; MEC 19, p. 105]. There are about 100 cannabinoids in cannabis, as well as many aromatic molecules (terpenes), which are also found in aromatic herbs that are part of the pharmacopoeia and are therefore also studied by medical research. The therapeutic properties of cannabis are attributed to the "surrounding effect" of these aromatic molecules in combination with cannabinoids. In the conditions that govern its medical use, cannabis is therefore prescribed for the treatment of pain, depression, anxiety, addiction, epilepsy and bacterial infections, conditions for which its mechanisms of action are not perfectly known [RUS 11, p. 163].

Therapeutic cannabis on the Internet

The fact that cannabis is still illegal in many nation-states but that it contains a large number of molecules that are of interest to medical research fuels strong discursive activity online, on specialized sites and on socio–digital networks as a whole (forums, Facebook groups or Instagram accounts). The international scientific activity around it is widely discussed on specialized French-speaking sites, some of which propose gathering health information on the subject[7]. Beyond the experiences reported by some users on the use of the product, radical positions are circulating on social networks. Some arguments[8] present, for example, cannabis as a panacea. In the eyes of some of the most radical followers of this alternative medicine, its historical ban by governments is an action made to the benefit of the drug manufacturers who distribute their own molecules, which are less effective but more profitable. Finally, it should be noted that commercial actors are already offering "well-being" products based on hemp (or hemp seed), taking advantage of the confusion between the legal cannabis varieties (cultivated for its fibers, but low in cannabinoids) from which they manufacture their products, and the varieties of therapeutic cannabis (rich in cannabinoids) that are currently illegal in France, both for production and importation outside of medical research.

Box 7.1. *Historical perspective on therapeutic cannabis. Links to the Internet and social media*

---

7 https://www.newsweed.fr/categ/sante/ or https://lecannabiste.com/category/medical/.

8 Such as the one presented in the documentary *Run From the Cure – The Rick Simpson Story* by Christian Laurette in 2008.

7.4.1. *Expertise and the online health community*

To understand the role of expertise and experts in communities dealing with online health, it is useful to look at the functions of the different platforms (and therefore their community management policies) on which they are found. It can be assumed that the primary function of the platform is to host the community, or at least part of its exchanges. The users of these platforms meet two main objectives: searching for information and sharing information, both practical and theoretical. These exchanges may have an affective dimension, or even a compassionate and supportive aim, but where expertise becomes an issue, particularly in terms of organization, it is when there is an exchange of information that can lead to the orientation of care behaviors [LEV 13, p. 3]. The forums as a whole enable the dissemination of information to the general public, as well as specialized information [PAG 11, p. 41]. It is this second dimension that reveals the need to take into account the nature, as well as the origin, of the experts who express themselves there, as well as the methods that allow such expertise to gain legitimacy.

Max Weber distinguishes three criteria of legitimacy in scholarship and politics: "charismatic", linked to the personal authority of a chief; "traditional", which comes from customs and traditions; and "rational-legal", where legitimacy comes from respect for laws and their expressions. What interests us here, therefore, is essentially the third criterion, where legitimacy derives from the respect of laws and their expressions [WEB 13, p. 126]. What interests us is essentially the third criterion, where legitimacy derives from the relation to a certain rationality, *in extensor* to a logical reasoning. The processes of legitimation of expertise thus derive from mediation processes leading to a rational validation of knowledge. This validation then follows from the attitude of the other actors in the space where these processes take place. This space must allow the necessary conditions for reasoned and reasonable argumentation to take place, without any power of coercion. These spaces of mediation, which can obviously be training institutions (universities, *grandes écoles*, etc.) or companies, can also be found in online spaces. As a result, the mode of legitimation of expertise is defined in part by the space in which it takes place and therefore by the nature of its protagonists and their relationships. From this perspective, online health communities can be actors in these processes of legitimizing expertise.

We distinguish the types of expertise according to their logic of recognition, spaces of expression and modes of legitimation. The "institutional medical" mode of legitimation indicates conformity to the legitimation devices specific to the health authority, in particular academic and clinical research. The "associative institutional" mode indicates a legitimation process taking place in autonomous organizations, but whose legal existence is linked to a legal status; these may be companies or associations. The "community" mode of legitimation, on the contrary, refers to the proposition that community spaces can support these processes of legitimation by seeing individuals participate voluntarily, without any legal commitment or administrative constraint, but motivated by a kind of cultural, affective or goal proximity.

Table 7.1 shows an initial typologization of expertise. The categories in this table refer to most of the expertise described in the literature and that can be mobilized for social issues in the health field. The first column provides information on the origin of the expertise (the *training* of the expert as such), the second sets out the areas in which they are expressed and the third indicates where the legitimacy of this expertise comes from at the time it appears as such.

The academic and technical–professional categories refer to the classic figures of the expert, coming from a training course and then possibly integrated into a professional body, from which they can also draw recognition. The modes of legitimation of these types of expertise are those that could be described as classical, since they are already recognized in society for their integration in public decisions.

It is in the description of experiential expertise that another mode of legitimation begins to emerge, one that is peer-based and not dependent on a hierarchical organization. This type of expertise develops through the experience of various situations and is recognized as such by the interlocutors who take part in the discussion and who approve the empirical path that led to the conclusions put forward. It is understandable that this type of expertise has a radically different nature from the first two in that it can be disconnected from any academic anchoring. It is legitimized by its peers thanks to the procedural path that constitutes it and that it allows us to see.

Lay expertise, on the contrary, which stems from the experiential, is by definition more related to a specific field. The lay is opposed to the sacred, so it is here the idea that sacredness comes from institutionalized knowledge. Consequently, experiential immanence will articulate, or even oppose, the institutional transcendence of expert information, which can only be "top-down" and unquestionable. Lay expertise implies then the positioning of an individual at the forefront of a field of knowledge that their training and preliminary knowledge leaves them outside, but for which they have been self-taught. This learning must be sufficiently complete to meet certain requirements specific to the qualification of expert, which we will see in section 7.5 describing the validation of expertise. This term therefore takes on a very broad meaning; we are not confining it to patients whose expertise is legitimized by the healthcare institution, and we would point out that it also stems from community legitimation processes, which can be found, in particular, in online communities dealing with health issues.

Type of expertise	Mode of recognition	Space for expression	Primary legitimation
Academic	Diplomas, research career, compartmentalized to the fields in which the subject is trained	Agencies, media, reports, conferences, profession, public debate	Medical institution
Technical–professional	Career steps, work experience	Professional environment, agencies, reports, media, public debate	Medical institution
Experimental	A narrative of experiences (professional or everyday life) that constitutes a peer-recognized structure	Professional environment, communities of interest or practice, life stories, media	Institutional, associative or community-based
Lay	Personal experience of the subject, outside of a career or academic recognition	Medical community, communities of interest or practice, forums, blogs	Community first, then medical institutional
Warm	Proximity, capacity to explain technical terms, to popularize	Discussion forums, workshops, fab lab, communities of interest or practice	Community
Citizen	Union, linked to the struggle and to movements of claims. It expresses itself in the face of practices perceived as illegitimate but legal.	Citizen mobilization, public meetings, public debate	Institutional association
Collective	Close to the citizen. Resulting from the number of actors who discuss the same subject	Forums, workshops, fab lab, communities of interest or practice, public debate	Institutional association
Community	Claimed by communities of practice, of interest or epistemic communities. Involves a compartmentalization of the rest of society	Discussion forums, workshops, fab lab, communities of interest or practice	Community

Table 7.1. *Types of expertise, origins, spaces of expression and main modes of legitimation*

The proximity expertise of the "warm" experts [WYA 05, p. 201] is qualified by making scientific information accessible. The aim is to popularize it, as well as to facilitate access to it. The legitimation of this expertise comes from the recognition of its translation action (from a technical language level to a more common language or information disseminated in a foreign language) within a group and to allow each member to learn.

Citizen and collective expertise have in common that they come from associations of individuals, linked by a legally recognized organization. The spaces of expressive pressure can therefore be any public meeting or online discussion that would appeal to the memory of a professional body, uses or citizen positions, essentially related to public health issues. Collective expertise implies a legitimation that results from a mediation process taking place within a collective that may be independent of a legal structure. Moreover, it encompasses, without enclosing it, community expertise.

Community expertise, resulting from legitimation processes internal to the community, particularly online, is manifested in relation to interests that are specific to the community, or relevant to the very nature of the community link. The community expertise of therapeutic cannabis users, legitimated by the internal mediation processes of their forums, remains the one of reference when it comes to the issues that concern them. However, the community expertise of some members of this community cannot be put forward where it could be heard, because belonging to this community is by nature illegal and so users can keep it a secret.

Community expertise also concerns epistemic communities [MIL 11, p. 13] in which the organization of knowledge is just as central. These communities are oriented first towards the production of new knowledge and then towards its use in the development of public policies. However, the reference to an external authority is less natural and thus reinforces the processes of intra-community legitimation. Indeed, there is no medical textbook that reaches a consensus on the therapeutic use of cannabis to which users could refer. Unlike recognized epistemic communities where knowledge production is directly integrated into policy-making processes [MEY 11, p. 143], there is no institutionalized use of knowledge production from online communities of cannabis growers or users of therapeutic cannabis as such[9].

9 It is only very recently, notably with the *Cannabis Use Survey* of Bastyr University in California, that institutional actors have taken an interest in these communities to obtain feedback on use and experience. The political use of the epistemic dimension of the community involves institutional (academic) actors, first of all, and also economic and industrial actors.

7.4.2. *Negotiation as an info-communication process for legitimizing expertise*

The diversity of media, places of debate and modes of exchange leads us to understand that the processes of legitimation of online expertise resonate with the mistrust of public institutions. Experts, whatever their career, find themselves in a situation of negotiating their position as an expert in each new expertise situation they find themselves in. For the expert, this is a matter of mobilizing a set of allies in the sense of Latour [LAT 06, p. 90] because she or he cannot act alone in the public debate. He or she (1) must rely on a collective (the community made up of the user-members of forum x, for example), and (2) must be recognized by some of the stakeholders, especially the public.

This prior community recognition then involves staging and displaying the expert's professional and/or informational and practical career path. A personal page, a blog or "culture journals" or "guides" for the forums we are interested in can participate in the legitimation of the expertise of a community member, in the manner of a CV. This recognition depends on what is known about the individual's path in the area of knowledge concerned by the situation. This form of knowing can therefore be the result of a display that can be consulted online. However, the logical and semantic construction of a proposal also enters into account in the understanding of the expertise of its sender. The legitimation of an individual's expertise then passes through these two aspects: his or her capacity to express his or her subject in a specialized language, on the one hand, and the visibility of the research approaches and methods used that have enabled him or her to formulate certain proposals, on the other hand.

7.4.3. *The legitimation of expertise or the production of a community consensus*

The position of the expert patient is interesting to observe. This is a patient who lacks the medical knowledge that specialists with her or his condition possess, and is therefore a layperson par excellence. However, can he or she compensate for the narrowness of his or her own experience by documenting himself or herself to the point of being able to challenge the expertise (also nourished by experience, but to a much greater extent) of his or her practitioner? How does the medical profession recognize the knowledge of the layperson? How can the layperson become an expert on his or her illness and on certain alternative treatments outside the health system, outside the health authority? Can he or she still be qualified as an expert in this case? We will see that the analysis does not focus on the aspect of rejection or circumvention of the health authority, but rather on a redefinition of its framework of expression.

There is essentially opposing expertise on questions relating to the institution of the expertise, as Robert Castel says about the mandated expert and the instituting expert [CAS 85, p. 1]. The instituting quality of the expert concerns her or his capacity to mobilize certain knowledge in a particular context (to the detriment of others) in situations where it can be used to propose a diagnosis or a solution. As an illustration, on health issues the medical world proposes a framework defined by epidemiological studies. As this may be indispensable for the question of the risk linked to drug use, this framework may be a bias for perceiving the effects of certain practices. For example, low-dose cannabis use could have an impact on well-being before having an effect that can be qualified as recreational. However, the epidemiological view of cannabis use (through the risks arising from use) does not, by its very nature, allow for the potential benefits of such use to appear. If official and academic expertise concerning cannabis is only built up from the study of subjects with behaviors identified as "at risk" by the authorities, how can it be given access to knowledge that does not only concern the risks induced by the use of the substance?

The institutional dimension of expertise is therefore central to the exploration of the therapeutic value of products whose use is controversial: what framework should be established to allow knowledge to develop around a prohibited use in order to see potential benefits? How should the related expertise be qualified?

In discussion forums where patient communities are formed, we can see stakeholders speaking as experts without meeting the criteria that would allow them to be classified as such. These are stakeholders who put forward a proposal on a subject around which they do not benefit from institutional community recognition or legitimation processes that are known to them by other users. The diversity of profiles, modes of pressure, and origins of the knowledge deployed there lead us to update our categorization of expertise.

The objective of this chapter is to show that the virtual community model [GAL 14, p. 268] helps us to understand the constitution of expertise. This model is presented as an emancipatory ideal of online forms of socialization. It is at the heart of the principles of community management. Community management is part of the digital communication strategy. It aims to optimize and enhance the interactions that Internet users have online on the sociotechnical dispositives of Web 2.0 or Social Web (discussion forums, Facebook or Messenger groups, blogs, wiki, etc.). In its main principles, it favors generous interactions (gift logic), reasoned and reasonable discussions (ethics of discussion) and an affirmation of all identities (logic of recognition). The idea here is to use these three social logics to develop interactions in the most fluid way possible, since developing interactions between Internet users means making them captive and available to advertising messages. It also means better understanding their tastes, consumption habits and social practices in order to accumulate data and build valuable user profiles for marketers. Community management, under the guise of marketing or managerial efficiency, is therefore associated with the promotion of a user-friendly and libertarian Internet.

Of course, the reality can seem quite different with the generalization of fake news, gratuitous polemics or insults under cover of anonymity. Nevertheless, at a time of Internet disenchantment [BAD 17], the ideal of the virtual community seems relevant to situating and understanding the phenomenon of online health expertise. Indeed, the gift logic, recognition seeking and ethics of discussion allow the constitution of a framework in which the processes of legitimation and delegitimation of knowledge can lend themselves to an analytical approach. This framework is particularly concerned with assessing the validity of shared information and its relevance, in a collective dimension, while taking into account the logics underlying exchanges between individuals in online spaces. We therefore propose a qualification of the expertise by taking these logics into consideration.

Expertise as we try to reduce and generalize it involves three dimensions that are related, but that cannot be sufficient independently of each other to understand the origin and qualify the expertise of an individual in a situation. These dimensions refer to the source of an individual's knowledge, which he or she will use to legitimize his or her expertise. We refer to these dimensions as academic, autodidactic and esoteric.

7.5. Framework for the community validation of expertise

The expert's understanding, in these negotiation situations, finally passes only through a negative vision of his or her competence, eliminating all traces of his or her incompetence. It should be noted that experts can reduce the field of their expertise by themselves by specifying the fields in which they are competent (in reality, those in which there is consensus). This is where the institutional quality of the expert takes on its full importance in the process of legitimation. We propose the idea of a pattern for qualifying an individual as an expert in a situation:

– if they are able to specify their field of competence;

– if they do not struggle when faced with knowledge that falls within their field of competence, that is, they know where to find the knowledge necessary to explain a situation, as well as to explain the limits of their field of competence;

– whether they can judge the appropriateness of using their skills and knowledge when necessary and intervene where their field of competence requires it;

– if others can attest to their competence in the field.

The ethics of discussion could be transposed to the expert in an ethics of expertise that would draw the contours of an ideal type of expert. It is then a matter of bringing together the stakeholders who express themselves by calling themselves experts or by being designated as such by other members of the community. This dimension requires a certain anteriority in tracing exchanges, which can constitute a bias for the methodical application of these standard ideals when they are missing.

To be constructed, the categorization we propose is based on the characteristics of the types of expertise in Table 7.1. It is the info-communicational aim of this categorization that interests us: the characteristics of the presumed expert come into tension with his or her environment, the other stakeholders and the empirical validation of his or her assertions. It is therefore the sociotechnical dimension that partly constitutes the environment of the expert we are studying: their capacity to mobilize traces and references to show the approvals of other members of their community whose expertise is recognized by the same provisions. These considerations inscribe our research on the sociotechnical mediation of knowledge in a reasoning specific to information and communication sciences.

7.5.1. *The three modes of legitimizing expertise in online health communities*

In this section, we will describe the legitimation process. We will detail what distinguishes the three modes of legitimation, and then what unites them. We will mobilize our fields to illustrate how these categories are mobilized in a proposal that draws on knowledge from diverse origins, ultimately different modes of legitimation.

First, (1) the expert whose legitimation is institutional intervenes in a field of competence in which he or she is recognized and has been trained academically. This expert can be opposed to (2) an expert whose legitimation is non-institutional or intra-community. We qualify this person *as an autodidact person with an institutional vocation* (see section 7.2 for definitions of legitimacy and expertise). His or her self-educated dimension does not mean that she or he is isolated, but rather that she or he knows where to go without having learned in recognized institutions, unlike one whose legitimacy is institutional. It is therefore this capacity to articulate the means (informational and technical) made available by the rest of the community that constitutes her or his expertise. To establish their legitimacy, these people demonstrate, within their community, their agility in handling newly learned concepts. Their institutional vocation is expressed by the fact that they can define a framework for understanding a problem, and then attach to it the appropriate sources of information. This practice borrows from empirical information research, which could be described as inductive practice. However, this search for information becomes a hypothetical-deductive approach to look for the right terms and presume good relations between them, and finally to expose the results in a clear way. The third type of legitimation of expertise is (3) esoteric (non-institutional) legitimation. The related expert has become so by his or her seniority in the practice in question. He or she therefore possesses knowledge that predates his or her attendance at the CSAI/place in which he or she expresses himself or herself, which he or she may have acquired in an autodidactic way, but unlike the latter, his or her construction is not displayed online on the platforms he or she uses. The esoteric dimension encompasses the entire process of legitimizing his or her expertise. This expertise comes from an ancient, insider practice that remains secret until it is claimed, either because it is simply not known to other actors, or because it was literally kept secret to protect oneself from the police. This expert will offer his or her own experience and insider references to shed light on the understanding of a problem and provide a solution. The legitimacy of his or her expertise can then only come from the recognition by the rest of the community in which he or she participates (through facts that may not be known at first glance, linked to previous relationships with other experts) and through assertions that can be tested and validated empirically by this same community, through which his or her legitimacy is built or reinforced.

The following excerpts[10] do not deal directly with health issues, but illustrate the three modes of legitimizing expertise in a single contribution. It is the response of one member to another, which leads him or her to assert his or her expertise in a hybrid legitimation process between the different forms. The first excerpt shows that the speaker claims to have a certain expertise whose legitimacy comes from his or her training:

> I'm trained as a scientist, and frankly a lot of the stuff I read on the Web irritates me. In fertilizers, some people will tell you that you need potassium instead, as was the fashion at one time, and potash at another …

The first sentence explicitly refers to scientific training, related to academic training, and borrows from institutional legitimation. The second part refers to what is said in the closed environment of cannabis growers and thus puts forward a

10 Example of the use of different modes of legitimation of expertise in a thread excerpt concerning the quality of a (self-)production of cannabis in a biological culture.

relationship with the insiders, proper to *esoteric* legitimation. The next part makes the link between what is said in the closed environment of the growers and what one of the members can do within these spaces, in the self-taught dimension:

> And we are satisfied with the guesstimations and the technical–commercial arguments of the manufacturers. On my former account I had written a tutorial proposal on mycorrhizae, and I explained, based on scientific publications, why it makes no sense in the context of our cultures.

The rest of the paper highlights a reasoning that illustrates the author's ability to use information and the resources at his or her disposal. The *tutorial* refers to a guide developed by a member of the community and made available to others. It is therefore the means of the forum, *in extenso* the community, that allow its users to organize their search for information and its availability to other members. The members of these communities then share their points of view and make proposals for transformation or consumption techniques that are discussed, improved and made available to other members in an index.

7.5.2. *Articulation of forms of expertise in the context of digital society*

The distinction of expertise is as much about the distinction of the practices observed. The expert whose legitimation is *institutional* will thus be enriched, and also limited by the knowledge instituted in his or her field of work. He or she will be able to intervene in a clear-cut manner on a rather limited number of subjects, the very subjects for which the expertise of his or her institution is recognized as legitimate. The *esoteric* legitimation of expertise takes place when a personal experience is shared and then approved by the community. This approval appears when the community empirically validates the proposals, which have been formulated in terms shared by other insiders.

It is when one is interested in the *autodidactic* dimension of legitimation that one understands that these different modes of legitimation can coexist. The legitimation of the expert who forms himself into a self-education person by instituting problems can be enriched by an institutional academic education. The part of the knowledge that he or she acquires alone can be enriched by prior academic instruction, and reinforced or broadened by a related skill through practice. Likewise, the institutionally legitimized expert can always supplement his or her knowledge through his or her use of the information resources or information research methodology in which he or she has been trained, to apply it to a field of competence that goes beyond his or her original training.

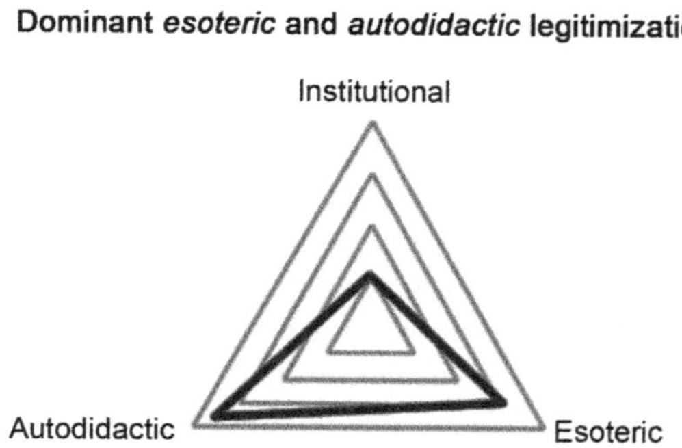

Figure 7.1. *Example of an expert profile according to its modes of legitimation: esoteric and autodidactic. For a color version of this figure, see www.iste.co.uk/cordelier/health.zip*

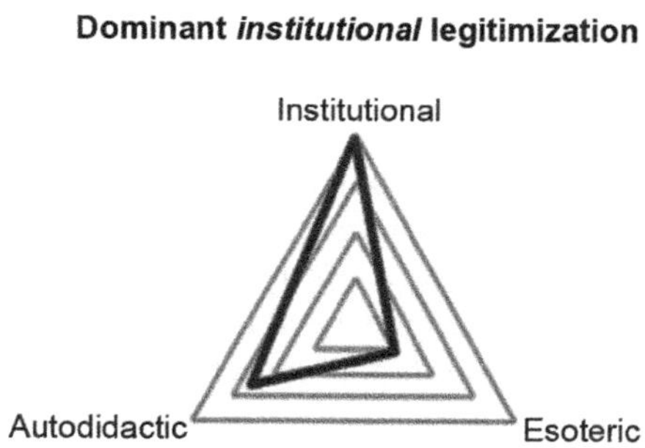

Figure 7.2. *Example of an expert's profile according to his or her modes of legitimation: institutional with little practice. For a color version of this figure, see www.iste.co.uk/cordelier/health.zip*

On the radar diagram (Figures 7.1 and 7.2) which illustrates the origins of an expert's legitimacy, it is immediately clear that the *esoteric* axis can be quite empty at the beginning of an expert's career and tends to grow later. The *institutional* axis, for its part, is not *a fortiori* destined to grow at the end of training, depending on the spaces we observe, since the practice (of a researcher), even if it is teaching, remains essential to qualify his or her expertise as such. To put it another way, the initial training of the researcher or physician (to cite examples of academic institutional origin) no longer plays a part when he or she begins his or her practice, and his or her seniority is translated in the *esoteric legitimation* axis. Finally, the axis linked to *autodidactic legitimation with an institutional vocation* corresponds to his or her capacity to institute problems in order to propose recourse to the appropriate field of competence. The latter is destined to evolve essentially according to the repetition with which the expert will institute or intervene on problems. It is the notion of "trace" that distinguishes the evolution of the *esoteric legitimation* axis from that of the (*autodidactic*) problem institution. *Fact checking* (or the empirical verification of information by the other members of the community) makes this axis evolve, which then takes on a historical dimension, when it is the institution of problems and the organization (online, and therefore visible) of knowledge in the field of competence that influences the axis of *autodidactic legitimation with an institutional vocation*.

The interest in building these profiles lies in the differentiations they allow and that are transposable outside online spaces. For example, they can illustrate the difference between a young doctor and a senior doctor: they have the same training, but it is the doctor's practical experience (in the secrecy of his or her practice) that is part of the *esoteric* dimension of our classification and that comes into account. This illustrates the importance of separating training from practice. In short, the *esoteric legitimation* axis includes a historical dimension, linked to the quantity or repetition of concrete applications of knowledge on diagnostic cases. It thus testifies to the solidity of the knowledge acquired through the seniority of the practice. It can be contrasted with the *autodidactic legitimation* axis, which essentially provides information on the expert's ability to orient himself or herself in the documentary and experiential resources available online and to articulate them in order to make a proposal for a diagnosis or solution. It thus concerns his or her capacity to institute, that is, to make the situation exist where expertise is needed by mobilizing the right resources. To make it exist, he or she must select the information enabling the creation of a framework for the diagnosis and sometimes mobilize the actors capable of providing a solution.

The axis of *institutional legitimation* exposes the depth of an actor's reflection on a subject or a situation thanks to methodological and theoretical tools in which she or he will have been academically trained. This axis makes it possible to continue to reveal, at least for the analyst, a difference between the layperson and the scientist by training without calling into question the expertise of one or the other. According to this model, a young graduate would only be represented by the *institutional legitimation* axis and slightly by the *autodidactic legitimation* axis: this would correspond to an individual possessing important theoretical knowledge that he or she would be more capable of reciting than applying in a situation.

This differentiation appears all the more indispensable since without it, the expert who was trained academically a long time ago would surpass all the others, whereas he or she may only very rarely have used his or her knowledge for a diagnosis or a decision-making aid. As such, his or her knowledge could not have been validated in the eyes of the rest of the community. This lack of involvement in situations that require expertise could then be a sign of a lack of competence or even ignorance, hence the importance of making this deficiency visible on the diagram.

This opposition then allows the *autodidactic person* who proposes numerous diagnoses, even if they are only sometimes validated, to be identified and qualified in terms of an expert in the sociological and, above all, communicational sense of the term. In this differentiation of the processes of legitimizing expertise, the role of the autodidactic person as an expert will have more resonance in the world around him or her than the one that we can assume is more educated, but who would interact less with their environment. We understand the challenge of differentiating these modes of legitimation: an actor who is able to better promote his achievements (by making them accessible to other actors online) will not benefit from the same modes of legitimation as an expert with the same training and the same seniority, who would not promote all of these same achievements. Finally, these diagrams are only interesting in relation to a specific field of knowledge, and our purpose is to insist on the difficult essentialization of a perennial expertise in an info-communication perspective.

To sum up, *autodidactic* expertise is legitimized by the transparency and the actor's display of his or her approaches to researching the use of the community's information resources, in short, what it has already legitimized. As for *esoteric* expertise, this is legitimized by the validation in broad daylight of the relevance of the actor's proposals, whose origin of knowledge is not known *a priori*. Finally, *institutional* expertise is legitimized by the actor's level of education, and therefore derives *in extenso* from the legitimacy of her or his establishment in the community. Among these modes of legitimation, it emerges that the *autodidactic* expert with an *instigating vocation* is the one who remains the most dependent on interaction with the other actors, and the one whose space for expression will potentially be the most reduced. This differentiation also makes it possible to understand expertise according to the scope of its influence: if it remains in restricted online spaces or if it is integrated or as a voice of integration in the decision-making processes of health actors or industrialists, for example.

7.6. Conclusion

Finally, after having observed the particular place of expertise in information and communication sciences, we questioned its qualification and role in online health communities. How can we recognize the *career* (in Becker's sense) of an expert among the members of these online communities? What can they have in common and where do they differ? We first came to propose a *pattern* for legitimizing expertise and recognizing its owners within these communities, in order to first bring together different points. We then categorized it according to three legitimation processes related to the origin of the knowledge of the experts observed. If it is of academic origin, it is institutional expertise; if it is acquired through practice, it is esoteric expertise; and if it is a capacity to search for and mobilize specific information in order to become competent in an area, it is self-didactic expertise. Each expert in these online communities is the result of these legitimation processes. Some of them derive from a natural authority, from their mastery of technical or theoretical points (institutional legitimation). Others derive this authority from the way they refer to past experiences (esoteric legitimation). Still others assert their legitimacy through their ability to search for, select and prioritize information to invalidate a proposal (autodidactic legitimation).

From a health point of view, the diversity of experts who express themselves in online communities brings with it a diversity of technical diagnoses or possible proposals. Members may adhere to certain proposals according to their beliefs, personal affinities or their own representations. This can be a challenge for the health authority, if it decides to express itself in online spaces dealing with health. It would thereby validate the expert quality of certain stakeholders by opening up a dialog with them in order to know and then support practices, as well as perhaps also to more effectively guide research programs on controversial subjects, such as therapeutic cannabis.

7.7. References

[BAD 17] BADOUARD R. *Le désenchantement de l'internet. Désinformation, rumeur et propagande*, FYP, Limoges, 2017.

[BEC 85] BECKER H.-S., *Outsiders : études de sociologie de la déviance*, Métailié, Paris, 1985.

[BON 16] BONNET J., GALIBERT O., "Organisations et savoirs : quelles médiations ?" *Communication et organisation*, no. 49, pp. 5–17, 2016.

[BOU 02] BOUZON A., "L'expertise en situation", *Questions de communication*, no. 2, pp. 3–6, 2002.

[BRO 11] BROCA S., KOSTER R., "Les réseaux sociaux de santé", *Les Cahiers du numérique*, vol. 7, no. 2, pp. 103–116, 2011.

[CAS 85] CASTEL R., "L'expert mandaté et l'expert instituant", in FRITSCH P. (ed.), *Situations d'expertise et socialisation des savoirs*, CRESAL, Saint-Étienne, 1985.

[DAV 04] DAVALLON J., "Objet concret, objet scientifique, objet de recherche", *Hermès, La Revue*, no. 38, pp. 30–37, 2004.

[EPS 95] EPSTEIN S., "The construction of lay expertise: AIDS activism and the forging of credibility in the reform of clinical trials", *Science, Technology, & Human Values*, vol. 20, no. 4, pp. 408–437, 1995.

[ETI 13] ÉTIEMBLE J., "Historique de l'expertise collective à l'Inserm et enjeux actuels", *Hermès, La Revue*, no. 64, pp. 102–105, 2013.

[FRI 85] FRITSCH P., *Situation d'expertise et socialisation des savoirs*, CRESAL, Saint-Étienne, 1985.

[GAL 14] GALIBERT O., "Approche communicationnelle et organisationnelle des enjeux du community management", *Communication et organisation*, no. 46, pp. 265–278, 2014.

[GRI 10] GRIMALDI A., "Les différents habits de 'l'expert profane'", *Les Tribunes de la santé*, no. 27, pp. 91–100, 2010.

[GRO 03] GROTENHERMEN F., "Pharmacokinetics and pharmacodynamics of cannabinoids", *Clinical Pharmacokinetics*, no. 42, pp. 327–360, 2003.

[LAM 17] LAMY A., "Mise en cause de l'autorité médicale et légitimation du discours d'expérience sur les forums de discussion en ligne", *Quaderni, communication, technologies, pouvoir*, no. 93, pp. 43–52, 2017.

[LAP 16] LAPORTE A., DUBREUIL M., JEAN-GILLES E. *et al.*, "Convier les citoyens des quartiers populaires : prendre en compte leur expertise et favoriser leur pouvoir d'agir", *Revue d'épidémiologie et de santé publique*, no. 64, 2016.

[LAT 16] LATOUR B., "Le prince : machines et machinations", in AKRICH M., CALLON M. (eds), *Sociologie de la traduction : textes fondateurs*, Presses des Mines, Paris, 2016.

[LEV 13] LEVY J.J., THOËR C., "Diversité des usages santé d'Internet et enjeux de communication", *Communiquer. Revue de communication sociale et publique*, pp. 87–106, 2013.

[MAR 15] MARICHALAR P., JOUZEL J.-N., GILBERT C., *et al.*, *Dictionnaire critique de l'expertise : santé, travail, environnement*, Presses de Sciences Po, Paris, 2015.

[MEC 19] MECHOULAM R., *Cannabinoids As Therapeutic Agents*, CRC Press, Boca Raton, 2019.

[MEY 11] MEYER M., MOLYNEUX-HODGSON S., "'Communautés épistémiques' : une notion utile pour théoriser les collectifs en sciences ?", *Terrains & travaux*, no. 18, pp. 141–154, 2011.

[MIE 10] MIEGE B., *L'espace public contemporain*, Presses Universitaires de Grenoble, Grenoble, 2010.

[MIL 11] MILLERAND F., HEATON L., PROULX S., "Émergence d'une communauté épistémique : création et partage du savoir botanique en réseau", *Connexions : communication numérique et lien social*, pp. 253–268, 2011.

[ORA 13] ORANGE V., MILLERAND F., THOËR C., "Profils et modes de contribution dans un forum sur le détournement de médicaments: une analyse diachronique des interactions", *Communiquer. Revue de communication sociale et publique*, pp. 87–106, 2013.

[PAG 11] PAGANELLI C., VIVIANE C., "Le forum de discussion: une ressource informationnelle hybride entre information grand public et information spécialisée", in YASRI-LABRIQUE E. (ed.), *Les forums de discussion: Agoras du XXIe siècle? Théories, Enjeux et pratiques discursives*, L'Harmattan, Paris, 2011.

[PES 07] PESTRE D., "L'analyse de controverses dans l'étude des sciences depuis trente ans", *Mil neuf cent. Revue d'histoire intellectuelle*, no. 25, pp. 29–43, 2007.

[ROM 08] ROMEYER H., "TIC et santé: entre information médicale et information de santé", *Tic&société*, vol. 2, no. 1, 2008.

[RUS 11] RUSSO E.-B., "Taming THC: Potential cannabis synergy and phytocannabinoid-terpenoid entourage effects", *British Journal of Pharmacology*, no. 163, pp. 1344–1364, 2011.

[SAL 15] SALMAN S., TOPÇU S., *Expertise profane*, Presses de Sciences Po, Paris, 2015.

[SIM 08] SIMONNEAUX L., "L'enseignement des questions socialement vives et l'éducation au développement durable", *Pour*, no. 198, pp. 179–185, 2008.

[SIN 08] SINTOMER Y., "Du savoir d'usage au métier de citoyen?" *Raisons politiques*, no. 17, pp. 115–133, 2008.

[THO 11] THOËR C., AUMOND S., "Construction des savoirs et du risque relatifs aux médicaments détournés", *Anthropologie et Sociétés*, vols 1–2, no. 35, pp. 111–128, 2011.

[TRE 02] TREPOS J.-Y., "L'expertise comme équipement politique de la société civile", *Questions de communication*, pp. 7–18, 2002.

[TRE 06] TREPOS J.-Y., "Savoirs professionnels et situations d'expertise", *Savoir, travail & société*, no. 2, pp. 7–18, 2006.

[TUB 16] TUBARO P., CASILLI A., *Le phénomène "pro-ana" : troubles alimentaires et réseaux sociaux*, Presses des Mines, Paris, 2016.

[URG 11] URGELLI B., SIMMONEAUX L., LE MAREC J., "Complexité et médiatisation d'une question socialement vive : le cas du réchauffement climatique", in LEGARDEZ A., SIMONNEAUX L. (eds), *Développement durable et autres questions d'actualité*, Éducagri, Dijon, 2011.

[VEC 20] VECERA L., GABRHELIK T., PRASIL P. *et al.*, "The role of cannabinoids in the treatment of cancer", *Bratislavske Lekarske Listy 121*, no. 1, pp. 79–95, 2020.

[VEL 16] VELASCO G., SÁNCHEZ C., GUZMÁN M., "Anticancer mechanisms of cannabinoids", *Current Oncology*, no. 23, pp. 23–32, 2016.

[VIG 18] VIGOUROUX-ZUGASTI E., "Experts et dispensateurs de conseils de santé en ligne : (en)jeux d'attention et de crédibilité", *Communication & Organisation*, no. 53, pp. 145–58, 2018.

[VIS 92] VISSER W., FALZON P., "Catégorisation et types d'expertise. Une étude empirique dans le domaine de la conception industrielle", *Intellectica – La revue de l'Association pour la Recherche sur les sciences de la Cognition (ARCo)*, pp. 27–53, 1992.

[WEB 13] WEBER M., *Le savant et le politique [1919]*, Presses Électroniques de France, Paris, 2013.

[WYA 05] WYATT S., HENWOOD F., HART A. *et al.*, "The digital divide, health information and everyday life", *New Media & Society*, no. 7, pp. 199–218, 2005.

8

Identification Metrics Regarding Lay Expertise in Online Health Communities

8.1. Introduction

The healthcare sector is currently undergoing profound changes, driven in particular by economic and administrative factors. First, health specialists are increasingly forced to optimize their practices and reduce the time spent individually with each patient [BOU 03]. As a result, patients are increasingly encouraged to take an active role in managing their medical care [STA 12]. Second, the generalization of Internet access, the abundance of communication devices and the improved performance of search engines have changed the way in which health information is accessed. Not only is medical information no longer reserved only for specialists, it has also become much more diversified, particularly following the development of online health communities (OHCs). These communities allow lay users to organize themselves as producers of information, thus forming a "smart crowd" through collective knowledge sharing [FLI 10]. Consequently, in only a few years, the entire paradigm of creation and access to medical information has been transformed: publicly accessible data is no longer as easily controlled by a small number of institutional actors [STI 14], and the volume of exchanges recorded daily on these platforms makes any form of manual and systematic verification impossible. In this respect, many specialists question the reliability of medical information published on the Internet [NAB 02]. In a field as sensitive as healthcare, it is understandable that the control of information is a source of major concern, both for the medical community and for the citizens who consume this information. Nevertheless, we believe that OHCs provide a forum for discussion between contributors with varying levels of expertise, each with different but complementary skills in institutional

---

Chapter written by Damien DE MEYERE.

medical information. Hence, we are interested in the notion of expertise within OHCs and study the different updates of the figure of the lay expert within them.

The study of expertise and roles within online communities in general is not new, but, to the best of our knowledge, most work analyzes the interactions between different actors in a community by relying on activity logs, that is, time-stamped records of actions (content creation, response, like, share, etc.) taken on the platform, thus modeling interactions in the form of links between one or more nodes to highlight cohesive sub-groups of users, and study their evolution. The objects of study are in particular emails exchanged in companies [CAM 03], forums specializing in IT support [TOR 10, ZHA 07] or platforms structured in the form of questions and answers [PAL 10]. However, most of this research does not take into account the semantic content of interactions. Indeed, analyzing such a large volume of textual data represents a major challenge for the researcher, as the textual nature and the weakly structured nature of the messages make their exploitation on a large scale more difficult. Hence, existing work that focuses on the content of exchanges and not only on the types of activities that take place within them is based on manual and targeted content analysis, which is necessarily limited in scope [MAL 05]. Within this framework, our approach aims to link this textual content to a certain form of expertise by taking advantage of the potentialities of the computer tool and, in particular, the techniques of natural language processing (NLP). To do so, we are developing and testing a set of metrics and determining the extent to which they can be used to highlight a particular profile of lay expertise on the "Health" forums of Doctissimo – a site that is very popular in the French-speaking world.

This chapter is structured as follows. First, in section 8.2, we will look more closely at the issue of expertise within online communities and the resulting information management issues. Then, in section 8.3, we will present various indicators that can potentially be used to uncover certain expertise profiles. Finally, we will look at the results produced by our various indicators and see to what extent they provide us with a more precise vision of the various forms of appropriation of the register of lay expertise within the OHCs (sections 8.4 and 8.5).

NATURAL LANGUAGE PROCESSING.–

Natural language processing (NLP) is a discipline that lies at the crossroads between linguistics and computer science. Its objective is to develop a set of algorithms, statistical models and linguistic resources that make it possible to process human language, whether written or spoken, using computer software. Search engines, virtual personal assistants installed on cell phones and question answering systems are good examples of the omnipresence of NLP technologies in our daily lives. For each of these programs, structuring information is essential: whether it is extracting dates or schedules from emails to plan an event or identifying the actions to be taken following a voice command, content analysis is at the heart of this type of application.

8.2. Online health information and the notion of expertise

As we have just seen, collaborative web technologies offer unprecedented potential in terms of transmitting lay knowledge. Despite their controversial nature, OHCs bring together non-specialist users sharing knowledge related to their experiences with health issues. This recent focus on the patient experience through digital platforms has probably served as a basis for initiatives aimed at further integrating the patient into the care pathway, and gradually moving away from a paternalistic model where only the specialist is considered capable of providing advice [BAT 12]. Gradually, the traditional distinction between medical experts and lay people without any expertise tends to soften, and we gradually distinguish the clinical expertise of the specialist and the so-called "experiential" expertise of the patient [HAR 11]. The latter becomes an "expert patient" [BOU 12], eager to learn about his or her medical condition, and who gradually acquires a certain expertise on the basis of personal experience [ROM 12]. Individuals, strengthened by their experience, can then exchange and organize themselves into communities of Internet users sharing the same interest and/or goal, thus creating a sense of belonging that goes beyond geographical or organizational boundaries [PRE 00]. In contrast to the roles assigned in conventional organizations, roles in OHCs are not predefined, but are negotiated through interactions. For this reason, we believe it is particularly important to focus on this issue.

Despite the potential problems with the veracity of the information published on the OHCs, several studies have highlighted the following user expectations. First, it would seem that for a majority of them, these platforms do not supplant the specialist [STA 12]. Indeed, while OHCs are certainly used to obtain informational support, they are largely used to cover an aspect of health information that can only be partially addressed by medical experts: it is not simply a matter of exchanging factual information about health issues, but, above all, of sharing one's personal experience and knowledge as a patient [NAB 02]. Lave and Wenger [LAV 91] have indeed shown that learning from the multiple experiences of people in a community is an effective way to acquire a body of knowledge, which can, in turn, be used by an individual to understand his or her problems or needs and make decisions. For example, thanks to OHCs, patients can learn about treatment options, discuss them with their doctors and take an active part in managing their medical records [EYS 04]. In other words, the increased accessibility of health information would facilitate the process of self-identification and the empowerment of patients by helping them to make responsible and informed health decisions.

While the benefits of OHCs are not entirely disputed by the health specialists, it is also understandable that the quality of the information published on them raises questions. Huh and Pratt [HUH 14] also use the double-edged sword metaphor, with, on the one hand, a support that physicians can hardly provide in their daily practice, and, on the other hand, the production of information by contributors who, protected by the anonymity of a pseudonym, are placed on an equal footing in terms of credibility. On many platforms, the moderators' role seems to be limited to deleting advertising messages and erasing practitioners' contact information, which is a legal obligation, insofar as it is legally prohibited in France to make online consultations, on the one hand, and to advertise for doctors, on the other hand (Article R.4127-13 of the French Public Health Code). This legal prohibition suggests that a few specialists would identify themselves as such if they were to intervene on a forum, and all users, hidden behind a pseudonym, are therefore placed on the same footing in terms of credibility. Hence, in an attempt to shed light on the issue of information quality within OHCs, we are interested in the different forms of appropriation of the register of expertise on these platforms. Given the essentially general public nature of OHCs, it should be noted that our study does not aim to identify physician experts as such, but rather any user of the platform who presents a particular expertise profile that could be useful to other members of the community. In order to do so, we are working with an authentic corpus of interactions in French, presented in section 8.3.

8.3. Data selection and presentation

In the French-speaking world, Doctissimo is one of the most visited health websites, with almost 40 million monthly visits[1]. What makes Doctissimo so successful is its numerous forums, which have a vitality that is always very important. Created in 2000 by two doctors, Doctissimo is now part of the portfolio of a large French group active in audiovisual media; it is therefore not associated with an organization active in the medical world.

Within the framework of an agreement between Doctissimo and the Center for Natural Language Processing (*Centre de traitement automatique du langage,* CENTAL) at UCLouvain in Belgium, we have a large corpus of interactions recorded on the Doctissimo "Health" forums. The extraction of the raw data on which our developments are based consists of more than 22 million messages posted between 2000 and 2016 on 87 health topics. It should be noted that the productions analyzed were not collected in an experimental context: on the contrary, they are on the side of spontaneous written production, which has the advantage of reducing the paradox of the observer, insofar as the members of the community exchanged without the

1 http://www.acpm.fr/Support-Numerique/site/doctissimo-fr (accessed February 8, 2019).

intervention of a researcher at the risk of influencing the expression of their thoughts [HOL 12].

Obviously, the exploitation of such a volume of authentic data, even if it is the subject of an agreement with the publisher, cannot be done without ethical reflection about its exploitation. To this end, we specify that we do not have any private metadata concerning users, except for publicly distributed pseudonyms. Then, we consider that the textual exchanges to be the reflection of public behaviors, insofar as the Doctissimo forums are free to access [HER 96]. Finally, the users have all accepted the general conditions of use of the platform, which provide for the processing of data within the framework of a partnership agreement. From the point of view of our research, we underline that the tools developed under this framework aim to highlight types of behaviors at work on the platform without pointing to specific individuals. Finally, the examples and illustrations in this chapter are presented in such a way that it is not possible to identify the individuals behind the contributions.

8.4. Description of the measures

In an attempt to uncover lay expert profiles within our corpus, we have implemented a set of measures to characterize the users of the platform. These measures, calculated using computer programs specially developed for this research, are grouped into three main categories:

– metrics that quantify the number of actions taken on the platform. These metrics can describe individual user engagement or highlight the vitality of user groups within the community. As mentioned above, these relatively simple to calculate metrics are often used when analyzing online communities;

– metrics related to the content of the exchanges, which allow the intentionality of the exchanges to emerge. To set up these metrics, we use, in particular, text analysis techniques inspired by research in natural language processing;

– metrics that position users within the network of interactions on the platform. Indeed, through the use of the software, connections are created between users. It will then be a question of seeing the extent to which certain actions contribute to the establishment of a certain form of expertise.

8.4.1. *Characterizing engagement*

Several measures can describe individual user engagement or highlight the vitality of user groups within the community. Examples include the number of messages posted, the number of topics initiated and responses sent, or the degree of dispersion among sub-forums. Aggregating these data allows us to judge the platform's vitality and to get an overview of the types of uses that are developing.

In addition to the volume of participation, a user's engagement may be characterized by his or her tendency to initiate new topics or intervene in existing topics. A low rate of initiated topics in relation to the total number of messages sent would indicate that this user is more interested in helping other members of the community. However, a member of an online community who is perceived to be both receptive to requests for information and who provides timely answers to others' questions is likely to be considered trustworthy.

Finally, it may be interesting to look at the distribution of messages between different sub-forums and to determine whether users concentrate their interactions in a limited number of sub-forums or whether, on the contrary, their interactions are more heterogeneous. Our intuition is that lay experts will tend to concentrate their interactions in a limited number of sub-forums related to their personal experience.

8.4.2. *Characterizing content*

Although textual exchanges account for a significant part of the information published on OHCs, and probably the most visible traces of this collaborative knowledge production activity, few studies take into account the semantic content of the interactions. Indeed, while it is a new silo of information in which we can identify structurally meaningful roles, this data requires the development of new methods and increased interdisciplinary collaboration. In recent years, the capabilities for storing and processing textual data have improved dramatically, and research in NLP has seen a dramatic increase in its visibility through applications such as machine translation, speech recognition and synthesis and intelligent search engines. The analysis and structuring of textual content are at the heart of these types of applications, and we apply information extraction techniques capable of bringing out characteristics on the basis of the textual content exchanged.

A first way to characterize the content of the exchanges is to calculate the lexical richness of a text, traditionally defined in linguistics by the ratio (type–token ratio) between the number of occurrences (tokens) and the number of different forms (types). This metric thus makes it possible to quantify the repetitiveness of a text by measuring the number of different words composing it [COV 10]. At this stage, we cannot assert that a higher lexical richness is necessarily a marker of expertise. While we might think that an elaborate answer is necessarily rich from a lexical point of view, it should be kept in mind that the informal nature of OHCs and the thematic nature of the exchanges could have an influence on the rate of lexical richness.

Rather than focusing on the score itself, it would be more prudent to focus on the significant differences between one or more (groups of) users.

In addition, one strategy for detecting dominant themes in large bodies of text is to extract keywords. In order to do so, we have developed a methodology for automatic keywords extraction based on the log-likelihood ratio, a formula used to rank (sequences of) words on the basis of a specificity coefficient [POJ 18]. Without going into the details of the computer implementation, this measure compares the frequency of sequences of words observed in a user's production with the expected frequency, calculated on a so-called "reference" corpus. In our case, we compared the production of a user with the whole Doctissimo corpus. The result of this calculation is that words used by a user with a significantly higher frequency compared to the whole community will be characterized by a higher specificity score.

While these keywords allow us to complete the information given by the dispersion between the different health sub-forums, we believe that they can also be used to highlight users using a more specialized lexicon. Indeed, according to Clavier *et al.* [CLA 10], the use of specialized terminology would reflect a certain form of credibility. As users become accustomed to living with a pathology on a daily basis, it can be assumed that they acquire a more pragmatic approach to their disease, and that they eventually master the terminology related to this health problem. In this context, it may be interesting to calculate a specificity ratio by comparing the list of extracted keywords with those found in a specialized medical dictionary. We have defined this score as the ratio between the total number of words written by the current user and the number of words constituting a specialized medical expression. The higher this ratio is, the more the user uses terminology that is closer to specialized language, as opposed to users who use the platform for chatting, who are more likely to use everyday words.

8.4.3. *Characterizing the interaction*

Finally, a third interesting dimension is the way users interact within the community. In this framework, an additional indicator of a user's reputation can be the number of mentions he or she receives [HUF 07]. In computer-mediated speech, it is not uncommon for speeches to intertwine, and mentions are a strategy allowing users to make up for the lack of physical contact when managing speech turns. Address markers are then used to ratify the presence of a user in the conversation [HER 18]. On Doctissimo, it is possible to mention a user and to trigger a notification to the latter by prefixing his or her pseudonym with the character @. However, we have observed that many mentions do not go through this mechanism, which makes a good part of these actions invisible in traditional activity statistics.

Once again, text analysis techniques are useful for extracting user mentions within messages. We then obtain a measure of a user's popularity through the number of times he or she is mentioned on the platform.

Websites such as Doctissimo provide a forum for discussion between contributors with varying levels of expertise, each with some knowledge that touches on different areas and that can complement each other. In this context, crowd consensus is a criterion often mentioned in the literature to judge the quality of information published on OHCs [FAN 13]. Hence, we have looked how the information published by each user is evaluated by the community, assuming that a lot of positive feedback about a contributor informs us of the competence of the latter. For this research, we listed two types of evaluation forms associated with a username: forms of validation of a previously posted contribution (e.g. "I agree with you …") and acknowledgements (e.g. "Thank you for your answer …"), which we automatically extracted and counted for each user.

Another way to interact with users is to quote their posts. On Doctissimo, as on many forums, a contributor can indeed include a verbatim of a message posted earlier. In particularly long discussions, a quotation can make reading easier by reproducing a message sometimes posted several pages earlier: used wisely, a quotation is a simple and effective way to clarify communication. Of course, taken separately, the frequency which quotations are used tells us nothing about how they are used, and whether their use is indicative of a certain skill on the part of the user. This is also true for all the measures we have just presented. Hence, we will comment on the main distinctions that the combination of our different measures create in our corpus.

8.5. The multiple facets of lay expertise

We have just presented a set of quantitative measures that characterize the engagement of each user, the content of his/her messages and certain types of interactions between users of a socio-digital platform. In order to see the extent to which these indicators effectively highlight certain expertise profiles, we have established a ranking of the users present within the Doctissimo corpus for each of these measures. During this step, we noted that several users were regularly highlighted by one or other of our measures, but that the rankings sometimes varied considerably, which seems to indicate that all these indicators do not necessarily have to be used at the same time in order to identify the same type of expertise, but rather that there are multiple profiles beyond the figure of the "medical information expert". We therefore believe that all these indicators do not necessarily have to be used at the same time in order to identify the same type of expertise. On the contrary, they show that there is indeed a plurality of profiles of lay expertise. In order to pursue our reflections, we selected several users highlighted by some of these measures and manually read their messages with the objective of determining what type(s) of expertise these users made use of on the platform.

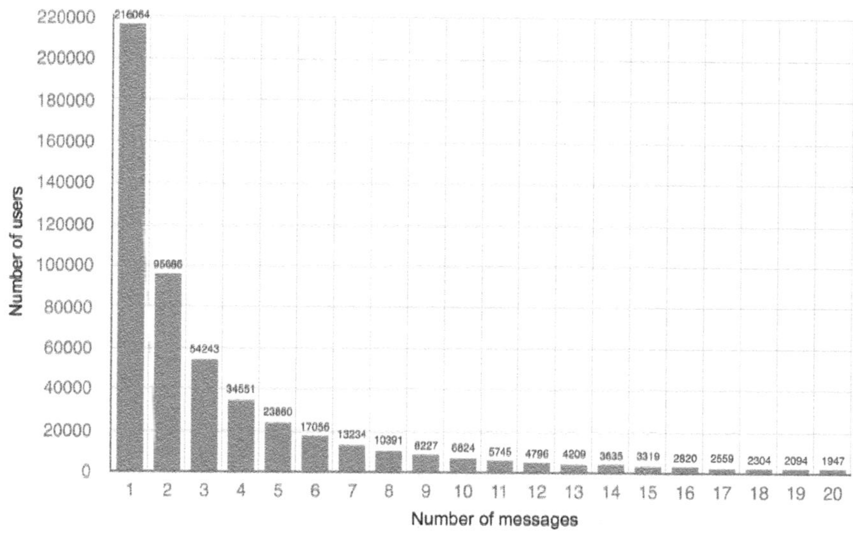

Figure 8.1. *Graph of the number of users versus the number of messages posted. For a color version of this figure, see www.iste.co.uk/cordelier/health.zip*

If we look at the number of contributions made by Doctissimo users, we can see that a limited proportion of users post a large number of messages, and that many accounts have posted only one message (see Figure 8.1). This finding is not surprising, since registration is usually done as part of an information search that results in a limited number of exchanges, and many users leave the community once their question(s) have been answered. It should be noted that this community structure, composed of a core of very active actors and a large periphery of users who are not very active, or are even passive, characterizes many other communities [FÜL 14]. From the point of view of user engagement, we have thus observed large differences not only in terms of the number of messages sent and the average length of messages, but also the subscription periods. The most striking is the low proportion of very active users who are loyal to the community over the long term. Conversely, we found that the most active users in terms of messages almost exclusively adopt the role of "responders". Nevertheless, we do not know at this stage what particular skills these users are likely to use on the platform. The size of their messages can vary considerably and is a reflection of certain user intentions. For example, some users get into the habit of writing long narratives based on their personal experience to reassure users who are sometimes very concerned about their state of health, while others tend to answer a question in a factual and rather concise manner.

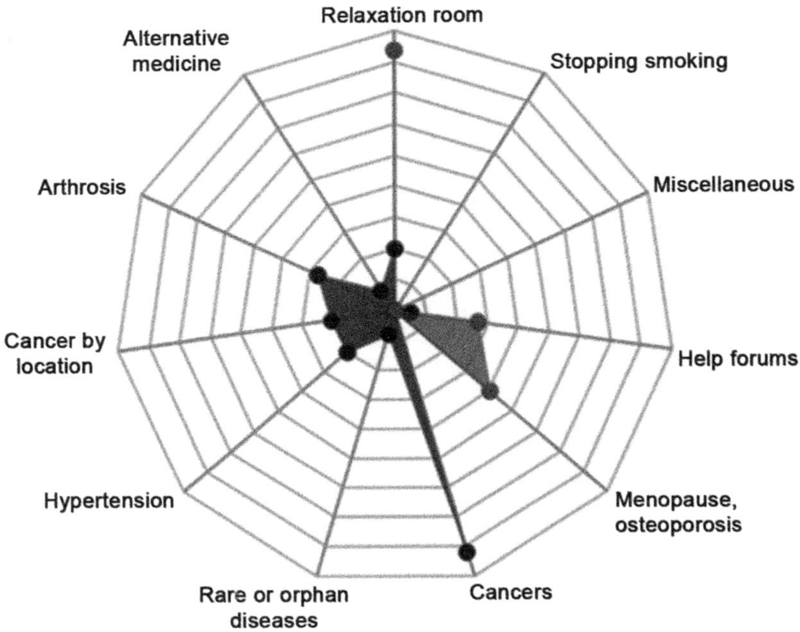

Figure 8.2. *Example of thematic dispersion for two users. For a color version of this figure, see www.iste.co.uk/cordelier/health.zip*

In looking at the dispersion of users across the different sub-forums, we found that most of the very active users specialized in one or more related health issue(s). Loyal members generally suffer from a pathology themselves and have subsequently benefited from the information available on the platform. As they gain experience as patients, they gradually begin to answer questions from other users and are less likely to approach the community with personal questions. These members bring a lot of information related to a health condition and support their statements with their personal experiences. Conversely, we have also noted that some users are more interested in the community dimension, for example by posting in the "Relaxation Room" forum, which is the section reserved for chatting and exchanges between members, or the "Help" forum, which deals with questions related to the use of the platform. As an example, we can take a look at the activity of the two most active users within our corpus. As shown in Figure 8.2, one of them is notable for being very active in the "Cancers" forum, while the second is mainly involved in the

"Relaxation Room" (i.e. the chat room), the "Menopause–Osteoporosis" forum and the "Help" forum (which brings together issues related to the use of the forums). Provided that the messages are posted in the right sub-forums, and without going into the content of the messages, it is clear that the two profiles differ in the type of information they exchange, with the former contributing to a few topics directly related to health, cancer in particular, and the latter seeming to be interested in the more community-based aspects of the OHC. As a result, users with an equivalent volume of participation may in fact adopt different behaviors: while one provides more informational support in certain health topics, the other may be more interested in the social and community dimensions of the platform.

In terms of textual content, we found that users with a very high lexical richness rate are generally those who participate in games in the form of message chains, and therefore do not provide medical information (e.g. the subject "ABC of Professions", which is not included in the "Relaxation room" sub-forum). This type of contribution, which increases user productivity and goes totally unnoticed with a quantitative analysis of the exchanges, illustrates the community dimension of the Doctissimo forums, which coexists with the informational dimension that we have already highlighted. Measuring lexical richness therefore helps us to distinguish between users who provide support on the platform, whether emotional or informational, as opposed to users who participate in message chains but who provide less health information to the community. In addition, we also found that more or less disguised advertising messages or spam were also present on Doctissimo. These messages very often include addresses of advertising websites, the name of a book or the name of a commercial product, as illustrated in excerpt E1 below[2]. Authors of such messages generally tend to refer to the same concepts, which act as keywords easily indexed by search engines, thus increasing the accessibility of their messages. As a result, these contributions are characterized by a particularly high degree of repetitiveness, and therefore generally have a low lexical richness. These messages drown in the mass of exchanges and can easily go unnoticed:

> [E1] A light stomach often causes fermentation. […] I manage by systematically belching until the feeling of bloating lies and the nausea disappears completely. I even wrote a book on the subject […] that shows all my tricks, including other internal exercises to get my digestive system to behave completely naturally and painlessly. I wish you the same.

In addition to the lexical richness, we were also interested in the words frequently used by users. Thanks to a keyword extraction algorithm that allows us to generate word clouds for each user, we were able to see that medical terminology was

2 These excerpts have been translated from French.

very present on Doctissimo, and that it was possible to identify areas of expertise that go beyond the categorization into 87 health topics initially proposed by the platform.

Figure 8.3 illustrates two examples of word clouds generated for two different users. Recall that the graphical size of a word is a function of its representativeness for the user in question, in comparison with the community as a whole. The size of the words tells us that one user differs from the rest of the community by the use of specialized terms such as "dyspepsia" (*dyspepsie* in French) and "colopathy" (*colopathie*), while the other probably speaks more about "Crohn's disease" (or simply "Crohn" – *maladie de Crohn*), as well as "extrasystole". These two users also use specialized acronyms such as "GERD" (gastroesophageal reflux disease – *RGO*), "UC" (ulcerative colitis – *RCH*) and "IBD" (chronic inflammatory bowel disease – *MICI*).

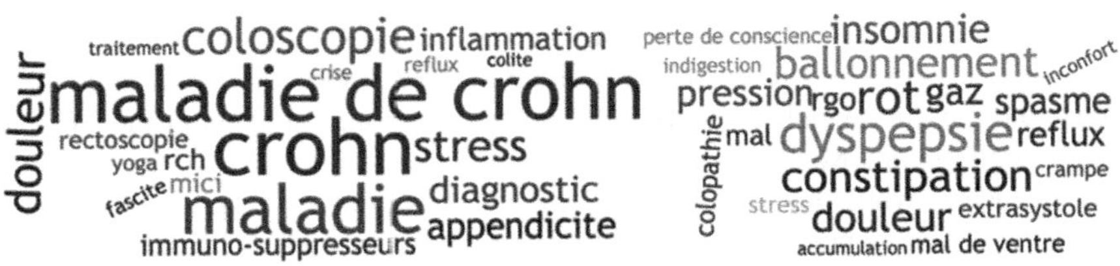

Figure 8.3. *Examples of word clouds generated for two users. For a color version of this figure, see www.iste.co.uk/cordelier/health.zip*

As we can see, the word clouds allow us to have a clearer vision of the themes that are addressed by users without having to read a large volume of messages. On the basis of automatically extracted keywords, we also experimented with a measure of terminological specificity. As a reminder, the aim was to determine the extent to which a user uses words close to the medical language used by health specialists. As illustrated in extract E2 on the following page, this measure makes it possible to highlight particular user profiles. In this case, the author adopts a particular posture that we believe is similar to that of the specialist (presence of a greeting, use of technical terms, requests for clarification, etc.), but does not present himself or herself as such. Our intuition was confirmed by the same user's comments elsewhere in the forum, as shown in excerpt E3. Moreover, it is interesting to note that this author takes a series of precautions and recommends consulting a doctor. This is not an exception here, since we have noted that suggestions to consult a doctor are particularly frequent, which clearly shows that the community does not intend to replace the specialist. On the contrary, the responses are most often aimed at explaining, reducing fears and preconceptions towards the medical expert.

[E2] Hello [nickname], // Tendonitis is usually accompanied by pain due to tendon inflammation. A pain that usually prohibits any strain on the inflamed tendon, so you wouldn't be able to run without difficulty. // Can you describe this "swelling" you feel? Is it painful to palpate? // A lesion will not stop your growth, however the practice of intensive strength training will; the ligamento-tendino-muscular structures need to dilate under the effect of growth factors to ensure optimal growth, the practice of intensive strength training places these structures under a systemic contraction that slows down or even prevents this dilatation. // It is also advisable in your case to take magnesium supplements for at least two weeks to preserve the muscle structures and help them to facilitate their contraction/decontraction movements.

[E3] (I practice medicine, yes, but my comments can only be for information, nothing replaces consultation.)

While the measure of terminology specificity allows us to highlight certain profiles that appear to demonstrate a certain competence, we are aware that the use of medical terminology does not necessarily mean that it is understood. A user may therefore post a large number of messages containing many technical terms without having a good grasp of the subject matter. For this reason, we combine a set of measures, which allow us to characterize not only a user's production, but also what the community says about it, that is, the interactions between members. Indeed, focusing exclusively on the use of medical terms risks penalizing users who do not address health issues in their production, but rather develop an emotional and relational competence. However, the latter contribute to the dynamism of the community by welcoming new members, participating in debates and games, establishing empathic relationships with members and guiding their peers in their search for information. These users may be specifically mentioned or even thanked by their peers, which shows that their contribution is useful to the community.

With regard to the mentions and evaluation formulas, we found that the most productive users are not necessarily the most recognized ones on the platform, even if the most frequently thanked users are, unsurprisingly, very involved in the exchanges. Similarly, some users using less medical terminology are regularly thanked, not for the medical information they communicate, but for the empathy they show. Even though it is generally the entire community that is thanked rather than a particular user, the counting of evaluative formulas makes it possible, as it were, to indirectly judge the quality of a user's contributions, whether they are more informational or emotional support.

Finally, our results show that the proportion of quotes made by users varies considerably: 58% of users who posted at least five messages never quoted any content and 26% quoted content between one and five times. Conversely, for one user, 83% of messages contained at least one quote. We observed an interesting habit that some members seem to adopt when quoting content posted later: it consists of reproducing a question asked and following it with either a request for clarification or a direct, rather factual, and understated answer. Quotations can therefore be used to demonstrate a certain capacity for synthesis and conciseness – two characteristics that bring the discourse of these Internet users closer to that of medical experts.

Here ends our overview of the different user behaviors highlighted by one or the other of our measures. By way of a summary, we therefore propose identifying four main groups of contributions on Doctissimo, each related to a particular type of lay expertise:

– **informational support**, which consists of providing information or advice in response to a question. Informational support may take the form of ad hoc assertions, which are expressed without citing the source, or knowledge from personal experience that is explicitly referred to or that arises from professional practice;

– **emotional support**, which is intended to show kindness, sympathy or encouragement for a situation without actually providing medical information;

– **personal narrative**, which aims to tell the story of a lived event, whether to testify (in cases where the author has experienced the situation himself/herself and wishes to share his/her experience), to support his/her words in the context of informational support (through his/her experience, the author is able to bring information to the community), and also to communicate news in a spontaneous way to the community's regulars (the author gives news following an experience related to the medical world; he/she then uses the forum to tell his/her story without explicitly trying to help a third person, even if this story can, of course, help other users);

– writings related to the **community aspects** of the platform, which bring together discussions that are not directly related to health aspects (e.g. moderator messages, discussions not related to health but contributing to the creation of a sense of community, family).

On several occasions, we have found that some users develop more emotional expertise, others more interactional expertise and others more lay expertise related to specific health topics. It would therefore be simplistic to consider health forums such as Doctissimo exclusively to be places where medical information is produced. While OHCs are, of course, used to obtain informational support, they are also largely used to cover an aspect of health information that can only be partially addressed by medical experts in their daily practice: it is not simply a matter of exchanging factual information about health issues, it is above all a matter of sharing one's personal experience and knowledge as a patient, and of getting in touch with people with similar health backgrounds, or even of creating a community around a health condition. Of course, these expertise profiles are not necessarily mutually exclusive, and many users mix these different skills, to a greater or lesser extent.

The popularization of collaborative web technologies has served as a strong driving force for the development of a wide range of platforms on which anyone can participate. In this context, researchers have produced a rich literature on the modalities of participation in online communities and the roles assumed by users within them. The common approach of all of this research, regardless of its theme, is to group together the behavioral patterns of the users of a community in specific functional roles.

It is true that the emergence of collaborative web technologies is bringing a new impetus to the nature of data available to researchers, since every action taken on a digital platform is systematically recorded. As a result, the volumes of data generated share many characteristics with what we now call massive data or Big Data. In this context, purely manual approaches are necessarily limited in scope and therefore often lack generalization. The risk of considering only the tip of the iceberg is, in our opinion, very real, and the inevitable errors due to human fallibility when analyzing a large volume of data manually must also be considered.

Faced with this influx of data, it could be tempting to limit oneself to a purely quantitative approach, for example by considering only the number of actions taken on a socio-digital platform independently of their intrinsic semantic value. However, we have shown that users with an equivalent volume of participation could, in fact, adopt different behaviors, and that it would be very difficult to see this through a purely quantitative analysis. Likewise, deep learning algorithms, which invoke the principle "the more data, the better the results", are most often like black boxes and therefore lack interpretability of their results.

Faced with increasingly rich, and also increasingly complex, socio-digital data, it seems to us essential to adopt a critical and multidisciplinary approach, combining the tools used in communication sciences, computer science, linguistics, statistics and other areas. If the capacities in terms of information storage and processing have considerably improved, we believe that the critical spirit of the researcher can be assisted – and not substituted – by these technologies, and that a fine analysis of social interactions within socio-digital platforms of any type cannot be without a good understanding of the methodologies and algorithms used, as well as the possible biases that each methodology induces.

Box 8.1. *Criticism of the importance of quantitative methods in health, cross-approaches of quantitative and qualitative methods in health in a digital context*

8.6. Conclusion

Collaborative web technologies have enabled the creation of online health communities that bring together non-specialist contributors. As a result, platforms such as Doctissimo now attract a significant number of visitors and contributors who, protected by the anonymity of a pseudonym, are placed on an equal footing in terms of credibility. Nevertheless, the volume of information is such that it is impossible to moderate all discussions. Hence, many specialists question the reliability of the information published on this type of platform, pointing to the difficulties encountered by users in searching for reliable information. Considering Doctissimo's health forums as a place for discussion between contributors with varying expertise profiles, we have implemented a series of quantitative measures to qualify, for each user, his or her commitment to the community, the content of his or her messages and the interactions he or she maintains with the rest of the community. We then showed to what extent these automatically calculated indicators drew the researcher's attention to certain potentially interesting profiles for analysis. An analysis of several highlighted profiles shows that there is a plurality of lay expertise profiles, which go beyond the expertise used by the health specialist. It emerges that some users develop more emotional expertise, others interactive expertise and others lay expertise related to specific health topics. If large-scale content analysis shows that there is a plurality of expertise profiles, these different behaviors would not only have been more difficult to identify through a simple quantitative analysis of the activities carried out on the platform, but would also have been very difficult to identify with a totally manual approach. In this context, the indicators developed are to be considered elements that can be used to detect trends, which must necessarily be confirmed by a more in-depth analysis.

In addition to their usefulness in terms of research, we believe that the measures presented can also help community managers in their practice by partially automating the detection of communities of expertise. From the point of view of the user producing information, it is possible to return a certain amount of self-confidence regarding his or her activity on the platform, to recommend content related to his or her fields of expertise, and to encourage him or her to interact with other users and thus avoid long-term fatigue – a phenomenon that community managers are struggling to counter. Finally, the identification of the types of expertise and the associated themes will make it possible to develop more advanced algorithms for classifying information, which will make it possible to find reliable content that corresponds to user expectations more quickly.

8.7. Acknowledgments

This research, conducted at the Social Media Lab of UCLouvain (Belgium), was supported by the European Regional Development Fund (ERDF) and Wallonia.

8.8. References

[BAT 12] BATIFOULIER P., "Le marché de la santé et la reconstruction de l'interaction patient-médecin", *Revue francaise de socio-économie*, vol. 10, no. 2, pp. 155–174, 2012.

[BOU 03] BOURRET C., "La santé en réseaux", *Études*, vol. 9, no. 399, pp. 175–189, 2003.

[BOU 12] BOUDIER F., BENSEBAA F., JABLANCZY A., "L'émergence du patient-expert : une perturbation innovante", *Innovations*, vol. 3, no. 39, pp. 13–25, 2012.

[CAM 03] CAMPBELL C.S., MAGLIO P.P., COZZI A. *et al.*, "Expertise identification using email communications", *Proceedings of the Twelfth International Conference on Information and Knowledge Management*, pp. 528–531, 2003.

[CLA 10] CLAVIER V., MANES-GALLO M.C., MOUNIER E. *et al.*, "Dynamiques interactionnelles et rapport à l'information dans les forums de discussion médicale", in MILLERAND F., RUEFF J., PROULX S. (eds), *Web social : mutation de la communication*, Presses de l'Université du Québec, Quebec, 2010.

[COV 10] COVINGTON M.A., MCFALL J.D., "Cutting the Gordian knot: The moving-average type–token ratio (MATTR)", *Journal of Quantitative Linguistics*, vol. 17, no. 2, pp. 94–100, 2010.

[EYS 04] EYSENBACH G., POWELL J., ENGLESAKIS M. *et al.*, "Health related virtual communities and electronic support groups: Systematic review of the effects of online peer to peer interactions", *BMJ*, vol. 328, no. 7449, 2004.

[FAN 13] FAN H., LEDERMAN R., SMITH S. *et al.*, "How online health forum users assess user-generated content: Mixed-method research", *Proceedings of the 21st European Conference on Information Systems*, United States, 2013.

[FLI 10] FLICHY P., *Le Sacre de l'amateur, sociologie des passions ordinaires à l'ère numérique*, Le Seuil, Paris, 2010.

[FÜL 14] FÜLLER J., HUTTER K., HAUTZ J. *et al.*, "User roles and contributions in innovation-contest communities", *Journal of Management Information Systems*, no. 31, pp. 273–308, 2014.

[GAN 15] GANDOMI A., HAIDER M., "Beyond the hype: Big data concepts, methods and analytics", *International Journal of Information Management*, vol. 35, no. 2, pp. 137–144, 2015.

[HAR 11] HARTZLER A., PRATT W., "Managing the personal side of health: How patient expertise differs from the expertise of clinicians", *Journal of Medical Internet Research*, vol. 13, no. 3, 2011.

[HER 96] HERRING S.C., "Linguistic and critical analysis of computer-mediated communication: Some ethical and scholarly considerations", *The Information Society*, vol. 12, no. 2, pp. 153–168, 1996.

[HER 18] HERRING S.C., ANDROUTSOPOULOS J., "Computer-mediated discourse 2.0.", in TANNEN D., HAMILTON H.E., SCHIFFRIN D. (eds), *The Handbook of Discourse Analysis*, 2nd edition, John Wiley & Sons, Hoboken, 2018.

[HOL 12] HOLTZ P., KRONBERGER N., WAGNER W., "Analyzing internet forums. A practical guide", *Journal of Media Psychology: Theories, Methods, and Applications*, vol. 24, no. 2, pp. 55–66, 2012.

[HUF 07] HUFFAKER D., LAI J., "Motivating online expertise-sharing for informal learning: The influence of age and tenure in knowledge organizations", *Proceedings of the Seventh IEEE International Conference on Advanced Learning Technologies*, pp. 595–599, Niigata, Japan, 2007.

[HUH 14] HUH J., PRATT W., "Weaving clinical expertise in online health communities", *Proceedings of the 32nd Annual ACM Conference on Human Factors in Computing Systems*, New York, United States, 2014.

[LAV 91] LAVE J., WENGER E., *Situated Learning: Legitimate Peripheral Participation*, Cambridge University Press, Cambridge, 1991.

[MAL 05] MALONEY-KRICHMAR D., PREECE J., "A multilevel analysis of sociability, usability, and community dynamics in an online health community", *ACM Transactions on Computer-Human Interaction*, vol. 12, no. 2, pp. 201–232, 2005.

[NAB 02] NABARETTE H., "L'internet médical et la consommation d'information par les patients", *Réseaux*, vol. 4, no. 114, pp. 249–286, 2002.

[PAL 10] PAL A., KONSTAN J.A., "Expert identification in community question answering: Exploring question selection bias", *Proceedings of the 19th ACM International Conference on Information and Knowledge Management*, pp. 1505–1508, New York, United States, 2010.

[POJ 18] POJANAPUNYA P., WATSON T.R., "Log-likelihood and odds ratio: Keyness statistics for different purposes of keyword analysis", *Corpus Linguistics and Linguistic Theory*, vol. 14, no. 1, pp. 133–167, 2018.

[ROM 08] ROMEYER H., "TIC et santé : entre information médicale et information de santé", *Tic&société*, vol. 2, no. 1, available at: http://ticetsociete.revues.org/365 [Accessed 8 March 2017], 2008.

[ROM 12] ROMEYER H., "La santé en ligne", *Communication*, vol. 30, no. 1, pp. 13–25, 2012.

[STA 12] STAII A., "La fabrique sociale : autonomisation et légitimation dans le domaine de l'information de santé", *Netcom. Réseaux, communication et territoires*, vol. 26, nos 1–2, pp. 55–76, 2012.

[TOR 10] TORAL S.L., MARTÍNEZ-TORRES M.R., BARRERO F., "Analysis of virtual communities supporting OSS projects using social network analysis", *Information and Software Technology*, vol. 52, no. 3, pp. 296–303, 2010.

[YAN 17] YANG D., KRAUT R., LEVINE J.M., "Commitment of newcomers and old-timers to online health support communities", *Proceedings of the 2017 CHI Conference on Human Factors in Computing Systems*, pp. 6363–6375, Denver, United States, 2017.

[ZHA 07] ZHANG J., ACKERMAN M.S., ADAMIC L., "Expertise networks in online communities: Structure and algorithms", *Proceedings of the 16th ACM International World Wide Web Conference*, pp. 221–230, Alberta, Canada, 2007.

List of Authors

Pénélope CODELLO
CRISES
University of Quebec in Montreal
Canada

Benoit CORDELIER
ComSanté
University of Quebec in Montreal
Canada

Damien DE MEYERE
ILC
Catholic University of Louvain
Belgium

Stéphane DJAHANCHAHI
CIMEOS
Labex LIPSTIC
University Burgundy Franche-Comté
Besançon
France

Olivier GALIBERT
CIMEOS
Labex LIPSTIC
University Burgundy Franche-Comté
Besançon
France

Géraldine GOULINET FITÉ
MICA
Bordeaux Montaigne University
Pessac
France

Anne MAYÈRE
CERTOP
Paul Sabatier University Toulouse III
France

Pierre MIGNOT
LERASS
Paul Sabatier University Toulouse III
France

Laurent MORILLON
LC2S
University of Antilles
Schœlcher
Martinique
France

David MORQUIN
Digital Use Delegation
CHU Montpellier
France

Ewan OIRY
ComSanté
ESG
University of Quebec in Montreal
Canada

Roxana OLOGEANU-TADDEI
E-santé
TBS Business School
Toulouse
France

Dorsaf OMRANE
LERASS
Paul Sabatier University Toulouse III
France

Hélène ROMEYER
CIMEOS
Labex LIPSTIC
University Burgundy Franche-Comté
Besançon
France

Index

A, C, D

E, H, I

Other titles from

iSTE

in

Science, Society and New Technologies

2021

DOUAY Nicolas, MINJA Michael
Urban Planning for Transitions

GALINON-MÉLÉNEC Béatrice
The Trace Odyssey 1: A Journey Beyond Appearances
(Traces Set – Volume 4)

HENRY Antoine
Platform and Collective Intelligence: Digital Ecosystem of Organizations

LE LAY Stéphane, SAVIGNAC Emmanuelle, LÉNEL Pierre, FRANCES Jean
The Gamification of Society
(Research, Innovative Theories and Methods in SSH Set – Volume 2)

RADI Bouchaïb, EL HAMI Abdelkhalak
Optimizations and Programming: Linear, Non-linear, Dynamic, Stochastic and Applications with Matlab
(Digital Science Set – Volume 1)

2020

BARNOUIN Jacques
The World's Construction Mechanism: Trajectories, Imbalances and the Future of Societies
(Interdisciplinarity between Biological Sciences and Social Sciences Set – Volume 4)

ÇAĞLAR Nur, CURULLI Irene G., SIPAHIOĞLU Işıl Ruhi, MAVROMATIDIS Lazaros
Thresholds in Architectural Education (Engineering, Energy and Architecture Set – Volume 7)

DUBOIS Michel J.F.
Humans in the Making: In the Beginning was Technique
(Social Interdisciplinarity Set – Volume 4)

ETCHEVERRIA Olivier
The Restaurant, A Geographical Approach: From Invention to Gourmet Tourist Destinations
(Tourism and Mobility Systems Set – Volume 3)

GREFE GWENAËLLE, PEYRAT-GUILLARD DOMINIQUE
Shapes of Tourism Employment: HRM in the Worlds of Hotels and Air Transport (Tourism and Mobility Systems Set – Volume 4)

JEANNERET Yves
The Trace Factory
(Traces Set – Volume 3)

KATSAFADOS Petros, MAVROMATIDIS Elias, SPYROU Christos
Numerical Weather Prediction and Data Assimilation (Engineering, Energy and Architecture Set – Volume 6)

KOLOKOTSA Denia, KAMPELIS Nikos
Smart Buildings, Smart Communities and Demand Response (Engineering, Energy and Architecture Set – Volume 8)

MARTI Caroline
Cultural Mediations of Brands: Unadvertization and Quest for Authority (Communication Approaches to Commercial Mediation Set – Volume 1)

MAVROMATIDIS Lazaros E.
Climatic Heterotopias as Spaces of Inclusion: Sew Up the Urban Fabric (Research in Architectural Education Set – Volume 1)

MOURATIDOU Eleni
Re-presentation Policies of the Fashion Industry: Discourse, Apparatus and Power (Communication Approaches to Commercial Mediation Set – Volume 2)

SCHMITT Daniel, THÉBAULT Marine, BURCZYKOWSKI Ludovic
Image Beyond the Screen: Projection Mapping

VIOLIER Philippe, with the collaboration of TAUNAY Benjamin
The Tourist Places of the World
(Tourism and Mobility Systems Set – Volume 2)

2019

BRIANÇON Muriel
The Meaning of Otherness in Education: Stakes, Forms, Process, Thoughts and Transfers
(Education Set – Volume 3)

DESCHAMPS Jacqueline
Mediation: A Concept for Information and Communication Sciences
(Concepts to Conceive 21st Century Society Set – Volume 1)

DOUSSET Laurent, PARK Sejin, GUILLE-ESCURET Georges
Kinship, Ecology and History: Renewal of Conjunctures
(Interdisciplinarity between Biological Sciences and Social Sciences Set – Volume 3)

DUPONT Olivier
Power
(Concepts to Conceive 21st Century Society Set – Volume 2)

FERRARATO Coline
Prospective Philosophy of Software: A Simondonian Study

GUAAYBESS Tourya
The Media in Arab Countries: From Development Theories to Cooperation Policies

HAGÈGE Hélène
Education for Responsibility
(Education Set – Volume 4)

LARDELLIER Pascal
The Ritual Institution of Society
(Traces Set – Volume 2)

LARROCHE Valérie
The Dispositif
(Concepts to Conceive 21st Century Society Set – Volume 3)

LATERRASSE Jean
Transport and Town Planning: The City in Search of Sustainable Development

LENOIR Virgil Cristian
Ethically Structured Processes
(Innovation and Responsibility Set – Volume 4)

LOPEZ Fanny, PELLEGRINO Margot, COUTARD Olivier
Local Energy Autonomy: Spaces, Scales, Politics
(Urban Engineering Set – Volume 1)

METZGER Jean-Paul
Discourse: A Concept for Information and Communication Sciences
(Concepts to Conceive 21st Century Society Set – Volume 4)

MICHA Irini, VAIOU Dina
Alternative Takes to the City
(Engineering, Energy and Architecture Set – Volume 5)

PÉLISSIER Chrysta
Learner Support in Online Learning Environments

PIETTE Albert
Theoretical Anthropology or How to Observe a Human Being
(Research, Innovative Theories and Methods in SSH Set – Volume 1)

PIRIOU Jérôme
The Tourist Region: A Co-Construction of Tourism Stakeholders
(Tourism and Mobility Systems Set – Volume 1)

PUMAIN Denise
Geographical Modeling: Cities and Territories
(Modeling Methodologies in Social Sciences Set – Volume 2)

WALDECK Roger
Methods and Interdisciplinarity
(Modeling Methodologies in Social Sciences Set – Volume 1)

2018

BARTHES Angela, CHAMPOLLION Pierre, ALPE Yves
Evolutions of the Complex Relationship Between Education and Territories
(Education Set – Volume 1)

BÉRANGER Jérôme
The Algorithmic Code of Ethics: Ethics at the Bedside of the Digital Revolution
(Technological Prospects and Social Applications Set – Volume 2)

DUGUÉ Bernard
Time, Emergences and Communications
(Engineering, Energy and Architecture Set – Volume 4)

GEORGANTOPOULOU Christina G., GEORGANTOPOULOS George A.
Fluid Mechanics in Channel, Pipe and Aerodynamic Design Geometries 1
(Engineering, Energy and Architecture Set – Volume 2)

GEORGANTOPOULOU Christina G., GEORGANTOPOULOS George A.
Fluid Mechanics in Channel, Pipe and Aerodynamic Design Geometries 2
(Engineering, Energy and Architecture Set – Volume 3)

GUILLE-ESCURET Georges
Social Structures and Natural Systems: Is a Scientific Assemblage Workable?
(Social Interdisciplinarity Set – Volume 2)

LARINI Michel, BARTHES Angela
Quantitative and Statistical Data in Education: From Data Collection to Data Processing
(Education Set – Volume 2)

LELEU-MERVIEL Sylvie
Informational Tracking
(Traces Set – Volume 1)

SALGUES Bruno
Society 5.0: Industry of the Future, Technologies, Methods and Tools
(Technological Prospects and Social Applications Set – Volume 1)

TRESTINI Marc
Modeling of Next Generation Digital Learning Environments: Complex Systems Theory

2017

ANICHINI Giulia, CARRARO Flavia, GESLIN Philippe,
GUILLE-ESCURET Georges
Technicity vs Scientificity – Complementarities and Rivalries
(Interdisciplinarity between Biological Sciences and Social Sciences Set – Volume 2)

DUGUÉ Bernard
Information and the World Stage – From Philosophy to Science, the World of Forms and Communications
(Engineering, Energy and Architecture Set – Volume 1)

GESLIN Philippe
Inside Anthropotechnology – User and Culture Centered Experience
(Social Interdisciplinarity Set – Volume 1)

GORIA Stéphane
Methods and Tools for Creative Competitive Intelligence

KEMBELLEC Gérald, BROUDOUS EVELYNE
Reading and Writing Knowledge in Scientific Communities: Digital Humanities and Knowledge Construction

MAESSCHALCK Marc
Reflexive Governance for Research and Innovative Knowledge (Responsible Research and Innovation Set - Volume 6)

PARK Sejin, GUILLE-ESCURET Georges
Sociobiology vs Socioecology: Consequences of an Unraveling Debate (Interdisciplinarity between Biological Sciences and Social Sciences Set – Volume 1)

PELLÉ Sophie
Business, Innovation and Responsibility (Responsible Research and Innovation Set – Volume 7)

2016

BRONNER Gérald
Belief and Misbelief Asymmetry on the Internet

EL FALLAH SEGHROUCHNI Amal, ISHIKAWA Fuyuki, HÉRAULT Laurent, TOKUDA Hideyuki
Enablers for Smart Cities

GIANNI Robert
Responsibility and Freedom (Responsible Research and Innovation Set – Volume 2)

GRUNWALD Armin
The Hermeneutic Side of Responsible Research and Innovation (Responsible Research and Innovation Set – Volume 5)

LAGRAÑA Fernando
E-mail and Behavioral Changes: Uses and Misuses of Electronic Communications

LENOIR Virgil Cristian
Ethical Efficiency: Responsibility and Contingency (Responsible Research and Innovation Set – Volume 1)

MAESSCHALCK Marc
Reflexive Governance for Research and Innovative Knowledge
(Responsible Research and Innovation Set – Volume 6)

PELLÉ Sophie, REBER Bernard
From Ethical Review to Responsible Research and Innovation
(Responsible Research and Innovation Set – Volume 3)

REBER Bernard
Precautionary Principle, Pluralism and Deliberation: Sciences and Ethics
(Responsible Research and Innovation Set – Volume 4)

VENTRE Daniel
Information Warfare – 2nd edition